TEEN PREGNANCY
AND PARENTING

TEEN PREGNANCY AND PARENTING

Annette U. Rickel

Wayne State University
Detroit, Michigan

HEMISPHERE PUBLISHING CORPORATION
A member of the Taylor & Francis Group

New York   Washington   Philadelphia   London

TEEN PREGNANCY AND PARENTING

1 2 3 4 5 6 7 8 9 0   E B E B   8 9 8 7 6 5 4 3 2 1 0 9

This book was set in Times Roman by Electronic Publishing Services.
The editors were Linda Lee Stringer and Barbara A. Bodling.
Cover design by Debra Eubanks Riffe.
Edwards Brothers was printer and binder.

Library of Congress Cataloging-in-Publication Data

Rickel, Annette U.
    Teen pregnancy and parenting / Annette U. Rickel.
      p.   cm.
    Bibliography: p.
    Includes index.

     1. Teenage parents—United States.   2. Teenage mothers—Michigan—
Detroit Metropolitan Area—Case studies.   3. Teenage pregnancy—
United States.   I. Title.
    [DNLM: 1. Parents. 2. Pregnancy in Adolescence. WS 462 R539t]
HQ759.64.R53 1989
306.7'0835'2—dc20
DNLM/DLC

ISBN 0-89116-808-7 (cloth)   89-2129
ISBN 0-89116-908-3 (paper)   CIP

To the memory of Lee D. Stein

Contents

Preface

This book was inspired by my work in the Detroit Teen Parent Project, which serves adolescents in the metropolitan Detroit area. As we grew to know the girls and to understand what they faced as young mothers, we realized we were obtaining a rare view of the world of adolescent parenting. It became clear that health professionals and lay people could benefit from such a vantage point. Thus, the goal of this volume was to present the existing literature in summary form while going beyond the realm of research into the actual lives of pregnant and parenting teens.

As a textbook, this volume will be useful in such undergraduate and graduate courses as Psychology of Women, Adolescent Psychology and Adjustment, and Human Sexuality. At the community level it is believed that a diverse population of health care providers, social workers, school counselors, and educators will gain further insight into adolescent contraceptive practices, pregnancy, and parenting as well as common problems faced by young mothers.

In addition, volunteer and nonprofit groups that have initiated special projects in the area of teen pregnancy (such as the Association of Junior Leagues, Planned Parenthood, and the Ford Foundation) will be interested in the findings of the Detroit Teen Parent Project.

The support of the Katherine Tuck Fund and the encouragement of the late Cleveland Thurber enabled me to embark on this project. Sincere thanks are also extended to those who assisted with the research and preparation of this volume: Jana Atlas, Christine Butler, Carol Gove, Julie Rummelt, Richard Smith, Elizabeth Thomas, and Joan Woodhouse. To Aretha Marshall, Director of Alternative Education Programs in the Detroit Public Schools, Asenath Andrews, Principal of the Booth School in the Detroit Public School System, and Mitzie Hoffman, of the Wayne County Intermediate School District, I express appreciation for their cooperation. In addition, I thank the Wayne State University students who served as peer advocates and the "little sisters" who enthusiastically volunteered for the Detroit Teen Parent Project. Finally, I am grateful to Peter Fink and his daughters Allison and Hadley for their helpful comments on the subject of teen pregnancy.

Annette U. Rickel

Introduction

It seems that everyone has known a teenager who became pregnant when she was still in school. Three or four decades ago a pregnant teenager was her family's problem, often solved by a hurriedly planned wedding or an extended visit to relatives far from home. Today, however, the rate of teen pregnancy, with its attendant physical and emotional health risks and personal and societal financial burdens, has reached a proportion that qualifies it as a significant social problem. Unfortunately, the adolescent population involved in this milieu of health and financial difficulties comes with less than adult maturity and resources to handle a task of adult proportions. This volume attempts to profile the teenage girl who becomes pregnant and the parenting choices and consequences that affect both mother and infant. The profile is based on empirical and qualitative information pertaining to teen pregnancy and its outcome.

Just how extensive is the incidence of teen pregnancy in the United States?

Chapter 1 begins by discussing teen pregnancy rates in the United States and compares these rates with those of other developed nations. Having determined the rates of overall incidence and of subpopulations, the chapter proceeds to outline personality and situational correlates of pregnant teens and to infer certain types of behavior as risk factors for future pregnancies. Chapter 1 also discusses the options available to a pregnant teen—from abortion to parenting. Implicit in any discussion of teen parenting are the pre- and postnatal risks to mother and infant as well as the risk for abuse and/or neglect of the future child. The facts and figures given in chapter 1 help illustrate the extent and proportion of difficulties associated with adolescent pregnancy.

The startling fact that many pregnant teens opt to keep and rear their babies raises myriad issues regarding teenagers as parents. Chapter 2 examines the research findings concerning both adaptive and maladaptive parenting patterns. Several variables are important in the development of adaptive or maladaptive parental behaviors, particularly those related to social supports, educational levels, knowledge of child development, and the availability of parent skills training programs. Among those factors that interact with these variables are the mediating effects of the girls' families and the teen fathers. Chapter 2 outlines the risk of adolescent mothers and fathers developing abusive or neglectful parenting patterns.

Chapter 3 focuses on the idea that infants at risk for developmental difficulty are found along two continua of causal factors. The three categories of influence that contribute to the continuum of reproductive causality are genetic, pre- and perinatal, and socioenvironmental factors. The continuum of caretaking causality is more directly linked to the interpersonal interactions of teen mothers and fathers with their infants. The research described in chapter 3 involves a number of caretaking concerns, including physical battering and other types of abuse and neglect among teen parents. There is also a discussion of the characteristics of maltreating parents and of intervention strategies to prevent abuse and/or treat infants at risk. Finally, studies are cited that appear to link particular maternal patterns of interaction with certain patterns of infant responsiveness.

Chapter 4 describes the author's Detroit Parent Training Project, which represents a joint program of the Detroit Public Schools and the Wayne State University Psychology Department. Begun in 1986, it is a longitudinal prevention/intervention program targeting an adolescent parent population in an urban setting. The project involves assessing the adaptive skills of pregnant and parenting teens, including social, emotional, and educational functioning. Peer advocates for the teen mothers intervene to provide supportive relationships and to help enhance coping skills. Other training experiences are provided to help the young mothers develop nurturing relationships with their babies and to reduce maternal stress. The program promotes mental health through early intervention. The methods and procedures are described, as are preliminary findings and results. As it is an ongoing project, data continue to be collected. The project team members include psychologists, teachers, paraprofessionals, social workers, and college student advocates. This model program is designed to be implemented by prevention agencies and school systems.

An important facet of the Detroit Parent Training Project is the role played by peer advocates for the pregnant or parenting teens. Chapter 5 contains a sampling of the qualitative data gathered by Wayne State University undergraduates as part of their assigned roles as peer advocates. The cases illustrate the types of social and educational interactions between teens and advocates and the advocates' views of the difficulties and rewards associated with the affiliations.

The first five chapters lay the groundwork, both empirically and qualitatively, for describing the risks and hardships of teen pregnancy and the types of interventions that may ameliorate some of the difficulties. More pressing, however, is the need to prevent unplanned adolescent pregnancies. Chapter 6 discusses models of contraceptive risk-taking behaviors and examines the literature regarding the possible reasons for teens becoming pregnant. Clearly not all teen pregnancies are unwanted, though they may occur more as a result of passivity rather than active efforts to become pregnant. It has been seen that sex education alone, family planning clinics alone, and school-based clinics alone are limited avenues for effective prevention strategies, although school-based family planning clinics in two metropolitan areas have been successful in lowering teen pregnancy rates in junior and senior high schools. It becomes clear from the information provided in chapter 6 that no one preventive effort is sufficient but that several appear to have potential for effectiveness given adequate staffing and funding.

While interventions at all levels, from prenatal care to parent skill training, are vital to reduce the physical, emotional, academic, and social risks to teens and their babies, perhaps future efforts should be directed toward a goal of primary prevention. This volume, which details the Detroit Parent Training Project, has achieved its goal of profiling the pregnant school-age teen and providing a model of mental health promotion that will encourage its use and expansion to further intervention and prevention strategies for alleviating this pressing social problem.

Annette U. Rickel

Chapter 1

Personality and Situational Factors Relative to Teenage Pregnancy

CASE STUDY: ANGELA

Awakened by her stirring baby, Angela checked the clock: 2:30 a.m. She was exhausted, almost too tired to get out of bed. She crossed the room to take the hungry infant into her arms and put him to her breast. She never dreamed it would be like this—night after night of crying and early-morning feedings. She kept meaning to catch up on her schoolwork, maybe even do her nails. But all she wanted now was to sleep.

Forty-five minutes later Angela climbed back into bed—another feeding and changing accomplished. She closed her eyes wearily, remembering the happy moments when she learned she was pregnant. She was radiant and certain that her boyfriend would marry her. Everyone was excited about the coming baby. The baby shower had been the most wonderful experience of her life—all that attention! And then came the painful breakup with her boyfriend and the long, difficult labor and delivery. Angela's eyes filled with tears. Her boyfriend had never even come to see the baby, and

Written in collaboration with Elizabeth A. Thomas.

she had heard that his new girlfriend was expecting. Wiping her eyes, Angela realized it was a dangerous topic to dwell on—morning would soon be here and the baby would be hungry again. What she needed to do now was rest.

Angela's story is similar to those of many pregnant teenagers today. It is estimated that 1 out of 10 teenage girls in the United States becomes pregnant every year, and many elect to keep their babies. Four out of 5 of these teens are unmarried. Many become pregnant in their early-to-mid teen years, and approximately 30,000 are under the age of 15. For young black girls, nearly half will become pregnant before they reach 20. The pregnancy rate among black females aged 15 to 19 is roughly twice that of whites, with 90% of black teenagers' offspring born to unwed mothers. Estimates of the economic burden shouldered by the U.S. government due to medical costs and public assistance to these impoverished families are in the range of $16.65 billion per year (Alan Guttmacher Institute, 1986).

Thus, teen pregnancy is currently viewed as a social problem of growing proportion. Researchers are seeking to identify teens at risk for pregnancy, striving to increase contraceptive awareness, and to improve health care to teenage mothers and their offspring. Many people complain that America's sexually active young people engage in early intercourse without awareness of the risks of unprotected sexual activity.

At present, U.S. females aged 15 to 19 lead nearly all other developed countries in the incidence of teenage pregnancy. Although not more sexually active, U.S. teens are many times more likely to become pregnant than their peers in Sweden, Holland, France, Canada, and Britain. It is important to keep in mind, however, that teen pregnancy in America is not a black problem. Studies show that while blacks have a higher pregnancy rate than do whites, white adolescents become pregnant at twice the rate of British and French teens and six times more often than their Dutch peers (Alan Guttmacher Institute, 1986).

Many believe that American adolescents, many of whom listen to highly suggestive rock music and view an average of 9,000 sexually suggestive television scenes per year, are ignorant of the basic scientific facts of human reproduction. For example, most teenagers mistakenly believe that they cannot become pregnant the first time they have sex, if they have sex infrequently, or if they have sex standing up. Thus, only about one in three sexually active 15- to 19-year-old girls uses birth control. Worse yet, some studies show that nearly one fourth of the young girls who become pregnant have been using some form of birth control, which clearly reflects a meager grasp on the adolescents' part of how birth control must be used to be effective.

To combat unawareness, such countries as Sweden and Holland make a point of "demystifying and dedramatizing" sex. In Sweden sex education is taught in the public schools to children as young as 7. In Holland the media play a major role in educating the public about contraception, abortion, and other reproductive issues. In contrast, public service announcements to inform Americans about teenage pregnancy have been banned by all the major television networks because the scripts contained the word *contraceptives*. It is the belief of some that Americans' avoidance of these topics is derived from the country's puritanical beginnings. Whatever the reason, American teens are getting mixed messages from adults about sex.

THE STUDY OF TEEN PREGNANCY

Because adolescent pregnancy is a problem of rather recent interest, there is a dearth of empirical information on it. Much of the research has been flawed methodologically, and results have been confounded by such variables as age, socioeconomic status, and the number of previous pregnancies experienced by the teenager. For the most part, studies of unwed mothers fall into three categories: comparison of pregnant girls who keep their babies with those who choose adoption, comparison of unwed mothers with other women in general, and clinical case studies of unwed mothers (Nelson, 1986). Traditional research has frequently rested on the assumption that teenage motherhood was deviant, and teenage mothers were seen as harboring deep personality problems that led them to illegitimate pregnancies (Dreyer, 1982; Juhasz, 1974). In contrast, others have found no difference between personality variables of pregnant/parenting and nonpregnant teens (Hatcher, 1973; Meyerowitz & Malev, 1973; Pope, 1967; Vincent, 1961).

Many fundamental research problems hinge on the failure of professionals to agree on what age bracket should be considered in the study of adolescent pregnancy (Hamburg, 1986). Preexisting conventions have grouped children and youth populations into groups aged 5 to 14 and 15 to 24. When addressing teen pregnancy it is evident that these groupings are inadequate. To overcome this difficulty, some have chosen a teenage sample of ages 15 to 19. This age grouping continually fails to meet the demands of teenage pregnancy research, however, in that increasing numbers of teens participate in nonmarital intercourse, become pregnant, and begin parenting prior to age 15. Additionally, and perhaps more importantly, 18- and 19-year-old females (among whom the birthing rate has declined in recent years) may more appropriately be viewed as adults rather than teenagers. Hamburg (1986) asserts that these young adults do not belong in the study of pregnant adolescents and offers the term *school-age pregnancy* as being more descriptive of the sample of interest.

Other age considerations in research include three distinct societal constructs of age: chronological, biological, and social (Hamburg, 1986).

Chronological age, based on one's date of birth, is the primary emphasis of industrial societies such as ours and typically overshadows both biological and social ages. It helps determine when one starts school, gets a driver's license, is eligible to vote, may legally drink, and so on. Strict adherence to chronological age when viewing adolescence is inappropriate.

Social age or social norms frequently dictate our expectancy of cultural or developmental milestones—such as marriage, birth of first child, and retirement. Violating the norms of the "social clock," either by being too early or too late, may result in stress for the individual involved.

Biological age is subject to vast individual differences in the developing adolescent. Females are typically 1 to 2 years ahead of boys in terms of pubertal changes, and within genders the normative ranges for pubertal changes are wide. Thus, Hamburg believes that the early adolescent may best be understood in light of his or her biological rather than chronological age.

Nelson (1986) believes that one of the primary shortcomings of previous research has been the study of pregnant teenagers as a unitary group. Because he believes there are psychological differences between girls pregnant for the first time and those whose pregnancies follow previous ones, Nelson opts to study *subgroups* of pregnant teens, without which he believes important psychological differences between the two groups are obscured.

From an intervention standpoint, Campbell (1987) recommends a breakdown of pregnant and parenting teens, as well as teens at risk for early pregnancy, into five subgroups: (a) school-age dropouts, (b) school-age students, (c) older dropouts (those who have been out of school for several years), (d) older students, and (e) graduated youth. Campbell believes that the needs of these five groups are vastly different, and he proposes that goals of intervention be tailored to each subgroup.

Because the study of adolescent pregnancy is still relatively new, these suggestions may greatly enhance our future understanding of the sexually active, pregnant, and/or parenting teenager, while increasing the effectiveness of intervention strategies. Additionally, the inclusion of longitudinal studies, looking at the inherent personality factors of a group of teens as they move through the various stages of adolescence, may better enable us to identify teens at risk for unprotected sexual activity as well as those likely to choose parenting as an adolescent milestone.

ADOLESCENT DEVELOPMENTAL OVERVIEW

A major concern relative to childbearing among teens is that teenagers themselves are still growing and maturing. Adolescence is a time of tremendous biological changes. In addition, in our society the early adolescent must make the social transition from a relatively sheltered elementary school environment into a larger, more complex junior high school, while shifting in role status from child to adolescent (Hamburg, 1986). These salient developmental tasks make adolescence a difficult time for many young people.

Puberty

Pubertal development follows a different course for girls and boys, with spermatogenesis preceding secondary sex changes in males. For girls ovulation is actually rather late in the female's developmental scheme, following adolescent growth spurt, attainment of early adult weight and height, growth of breasts and pubic hair, and menarche. While many view menarche as the final phase of female development, ovulation typically does not occur for several years after the first menses. Further, adult pelvic dimensions are not reached until an average of 6 years postmenarche (Lancaster, 1986).

Tanner (1970) suggested a five-stage model for adolescent pubertal development. These stages range from a prepubertal stage wherein there is no outward manifestation of change to a complete acquisition of adult genital and sex characteristics. In his system, menarche typically occurs around Stage 4, which, again, is relatively late in the female cycle of development. The average age of menarche in the United States today is 12.8 years (Hamburg, 1986). As mentioned earlier, boys tend to lag developmentally behind girls by 1 to 2 years.

The length of adolescence as a developmental timeframe has been increasing in the United States, resulting in the delay of adoption of adult roles by teens. Thus, although endowed with adult capabilities physiologically, today's adolescents are required to retain childlike roles for ever-increasing lengths of time. Hamburg sees this as affording teens many opportunities for too-early transitions into adulthood (i.e., early pregnancy, parenting, and marriage). Clearly, then, puberty and adolescent maturation embrace more than just the biological sphere; they affect a teenager's psychosocial and cognitive development as well.

Ego Development

Both cross-sectional and cross-longitudinal studies support the finding that ego development increases during the adolescent years (Loevinger, 1979; Loevinger & Wessler, 1970; Redmore & Loevinger, 1979). Loevinger (1979) has postulated various stages of ego development, each involving a characteristic mode of functioning. Each mode encompasses a composite of depth of character and impulse control, cognitive complexity, orientation toward others and self, and interpersonal style. It appears that changes in ego functioning take place slowly, possibly tapering off at the higher secondary school levels. This may have significance for the adolescent female whose interpersonal relationships and conceptualization of self and others will mature with age, thus affecting her level of responsibility in contraceptive behaviors and her capacity to adequately care for an infant.

Self-Esteem

Longitudinal studies of self-esteem seem to indicate that it increases with age, with increases noted during adolescence (McCarthy & Hoge, 1982; O'Malley & Bachman, 1983). This is not to say that such increases proceed in a continuous linear fashion, as decreases in self-esteem among seventh graders have been cited by some researchers (Simmons, Blyth, Carlton-Ford, & Bulcroft, 1982; Simmons, Rosenberg, & Rosenberg, 1973). Boys appear to respond to environmental changes (e.g., the transition from elementary school to junior high school), whereas for girls dips in self-esteem are related to environmental as well as pubertal issues. The lowest self-esteem values were noted for girls who had experienced menarche, changed schools, and begun dating (Simmons, Blyth, VanCleave, & Bush, 1979).

Self-esteem does appear to be linked to pubertal status among early adolescents. Tobin-Richards, Boxer, and Petersen (1983) found that early or increased development was a factor related to positive body image and feelings of attractiveness in males, though this was not the case for females. "On-time" girls were more likely than early-maturing girls to report positive attitudes toward their bodies. Earlier studies presented conflicting results for females, which appeared related to class differences. Clausen (1975) found early-maturing working-class girls to have lower self-confidence than their middle-class peers.

Koff, Rierdan, and Silverstone (1978) found evidence that the experience of menarche affects young girls' body images. In their study postmenarcheal girls, when asked to draw a female, drew mature women, whereas premenarcheal girls drew children. Nonetheless, Petersen and Crockett (1986) believe that the effects of puberty on an individual may depend on the personal meaning one attaches to it.

Conformity

Adolescence is a time of increased peer awareness and importance, when the need for acceptance and support from others is high. Females, particularly, turn to friends for emotional support and standards of behavior. While this phenomenon can be seen as a developmental milestone in some ways (e.g., the ability to form reciprocal relationships and emotional intimacy), it can also be detrimental to the teen who is overly concerned with conformity to group standards (Conger & Petersen, 1984). Petersen and Crockett (1986) suggest that along with increased libido and the need for emotional intimacy, a tendency to go along with the crowd is likely to result in early sexual experimentation and pregnancy.

Costanzo and Shaw (1966) posit that conformity follows a clear developmental course. For the most part, conformity has been found to be higher in early adolescence compared with pre-, late-, or postadolescence, typically peaking around age 13 (Coleman, 1980). Since early adolescence is a time of intense social and psychophysiological changes, it is understandable that teens look to others for support and acceptance. However, as they become more comfortable with themselves and their new social roles, the need for conformity diminishes (Conger & Petersen, 1984). Although conformity is viewed as a stereotypical aspect of adolescence in our society, it is not descriptive of all adolescents at all times. Additionally, teens are likely to model their peers in such behaviors as dress and taste in music; however, they typically internalize their parents' values.

Cognitive Development

Adolescence marks a period of great cognitive advances for the individual. By the age of 12 to 15, most individuals enter Piaget's stage of formal operations (his final stage of cognitive development), wherein one is able to carry on hypothetical thinking (Inhelder & Piaget, 1958; Piaget, 1972). One value of this to the developing teen is the ability to look beyond the here and now. With this stage of cognitive development comes the ability to foresee long-term consequences of one's behavior and to plan for the future (Petersen & Crockett, 1986). Such issues bear directly on teenage sexual behavior and pregnancy.

There is a general consensus that formal reasoning increases throughout adolescence (Keating, 1980; Petersen, 1983). Damon and Hart (1982) have found that cognitive advancements in the area of self-conceptualization and conceptualization of others, as well as the development of insight and judgment, parallel increases in the formal reasoning process. It should be noted, however, that the ability to extend one's time perspective and the capacity for self-reflection do not ensure mature judgment on the part of the adolescent. It appears that although the basic underpinnings for sensitivity and good judgment are in place, experience and motivation may be necessary precursors to their expression (Petersen & Crockett, 1986).

Just as there is a wide variability for timing of pubertal changes in adolescents, so is there a wide normative range for increases in cognitive skills. Despite maturing levels of cognitive functioning, however, periods of high stress and anxiety are likely to cause teens to revert to earlier, more concrete forms of information processing. This may impair their ability to improvise or make effective decisions when placed in novel or disturbing situations relating to sexuality, pregnancy, or parenting (Hamburg, 1986).

School grades tend to drop during early adolescence for both boys and girls, although girls consistently maintain better grades than do boys during this developmental period (Kavrell & Petersen, 1984; Simmons et al., 1982). Though some researchers have tried to link this with pubertal events, little evidence supports the hypothesis. Rather, it appears that more stringent grading standards as students advance in grade level may be responsible.

Other studies show a similar decline in students' performance on an encoding and recognition task (Carey, 1981; Carey & Diamond, 1980; Carey, Diamond, & Woods, 1980). Here steady increases in performance up to the age of 10 drop off during the period from 12 to 14, then pick up again at previous high levels around age 16. Again, an attempt to link the decline to physiological events of puberty failed when it was noted that both sexes show similar age declines, despite males' developmental lag of 1 to 2 years behind females in pubertal development (Petersen & Crockett, 1986). In contrast, Petersen (1983) found that cognitive test scores increased steadily during early adolescence, showing no evidence of disruption. It is therefore likely that social processes, rather than physiological changes, are responsible for fluctuations in cognitive abilities during adolescence.

Finally, adolescents appear to be subject to two kinds of thinking (Elkind, 1984). The first, called the *imaginary audience*, reflects the young person's belief that he or she is the focus of everyone's attention. This extreme self-consciousness helps explain teens' sensitivity to public exposure and reflects their inability to differentiate between their own preoccupations and those of others.

The second, the *personal fable*, relates to the specialness that adolescents feel. Young people are so certain that everyone is thinking about them that they gain an inflated opinion of their own importance. They come to believe that their problems, as well as their experiences, are unique. It is largely the personal fable that accounts for a teenager's sense of invulnerability (e.g., he or she may think, "others might become involved in an accident if they drive while drunk, but not me"). Both the imaginary audience and the personal fable remain with us throughout life; however, they are most pronounced during the developmental stage of adolescence.

Identity Development

Erikson (1959) described adolescence as the final stage of childhood. One of the tasks of adolescence, he believed, was the development of one's identity—a personal integration of values, goals, and abilities. Identity achievement elicits the feeling that childhood is over and adulthood is beginning; thus, it is viewed as the final resolution of the latter stages of adolescence.

Identity achievement is the integration of both personal and cultural values, and for most the resolution of an identity crisis is a product of both environmental demands and personal choices. When this is not the case, however, identity achievement is thwarted. For instance, *identity foreclosure* is a state wherein a series of premature decisions have been made regarding one's identity based primarily on the demands of others. Similarly, a *negative identity* emerges when an individual succumbs to environmental or peer demands and expectations that may actually run counter to the cultural views of his or her community. *Role diffusion* results when an individual is unable to make a commitment to any single view of him or herself and thus is unable to integrate the various roles he or she plays.

Erikson described the psychosocial moratorium as a period of free experimentation prior to the formation of one's final identity. During this stage the individual is able to try out various roles that represent the possibilities for his or her future. Because most adolescents have few social obligations requiring long-term commitment, the psychosocial moratorium provides a unique opportunity for sampling possible ideological or occupational arenas. Nonetheless, this period may be very stressful for parents who view their offspring as deviating from family traditions or life-styles (Newman & Newman, 1975).

Erikson's concepts of identity formation were used by Marcia (1966) in the development of a questionnaire to assess the status of identity resolution. He administered the questionnaire to a group of male college students. From their responses Marcia was able to delineate three groups of students: (a) identity achieved (had already experienced a crisis period and had clear occupational and ideological commitments), (b) identity foreclosed (had not experienced a crisis, yet demonstrated strong occupational and ideological beliefs), and (c) identity diffused (in a present state of psychosocial moratorium; commitments diffuse). Students in the identity-achieved group had somewhat greater ego strength than students in the other two groups. Further, students in the identity-foreclosed group demonstrated a strong commitment to obedience, leadership, and respect for authority. These students (who had not yet experienced an identity crisis) held occupational and ideological beliefs very similar to their parents and were found to have the weakest ego strength and most vulnerable self-esteem of all groups.

This study was replicated by Marcia and Friedman (1970) using college women as subjects. In contrast to the above findings, identity-achieved and identity-foreclosed women were similarly strong in ego strength. Additionally, in their 1972 study, Schenkel and Marcia found that the issues most salient to identity formation in women were sexuality and religion. This is in contrast to occupation and politics for men. Finally, a study by Toder and Marcia (1973) suggests that for women identity-achievement and identity foreclosure may be equally adaptive. Women in both groups demonstrated less conformity to peer pressure and reported significantly less negative affect than women in the identity-diffused or psychosocial moratorium groups.

TEEN SEXUALITY—"EVERYBODY'S DOING IT"

Sexual activity among teens has increased dramatically in the last 30 years. The Guttmacher Institute reports that adolescent females experiencing intercourse increased in number by two thirds during the 1970s. In addition, it appears that the sexual revolution, once limited to college campuses, has made its way through the high schools and into the junior high schools and grade schools. Unfortunately, the younger the teen engaging in sexual activity the less likely it is that contraception will be used.

Current statistics reveal that in the United States approximately 5 million adolescent females are sexually active. This compares with 7 million teenage males (Johnson & Rosenbaum, 1986). As would be expected, the rate of nonmarital coitus increases with age and is more likely to occur in couples who date frequently or go steady or when the teens think they are in love (DeLameter & MacCorquodale, 1979; Reiss, 1976; Sorensen, 1973; Spanier, 1975). Twenty percent of 15-year-olds report having experienced intercourse. By age 16 this proportion jumps to 33%, and by age 17 more than 40% are sexually experienced. In sum, almost half of all boys between the ages of 15 and 17 and a third of all girls in this age range are sexually active (Zelnik, Kantner, & Ford, 1981).

Adolescent sexual activity varies for blacks and whites, with blacks reporting age of first intercourse (15.5) nearly 1 year earlier than whites (16.4). Furthermore, birthrates for the two groups differ, although pregnancy rates do not. This implies that minority teens are far more likely than whites to give birth than to choose abortion (Zelnik et al., 1981).

Recently, public concern and interest have spawned the search for variables associated with adolescent sexual experimentation and intercourse in the hope that teenage pregnancy rates can be reduced (Jorgenson, 1983). Factors such as changing societal attitudes, family constellation, adolescent-parent relationships and communication, socioeconomic status, religion, peers and conformity, education, and pubertal and psychological factors of the teens themselves have been examined in the quest to identify adolescents at risk for early pregnancy. It is clear that these factors cannot be viewed in isolation but must be seen as working together to set the climate for the recent trend toward teen mothering.

Societal Attitudes

Attitudes toward sexuality in America have been changing since the early 1900s, resulting in greater freedom for both men and women to participate in nonmarital relations (Kinsey, Pomeroy, & Martin, 1948; Kinsey, Pomeroy, Martin, & Gebhard, 1953; Reiss, 1960). However, strong double standards toward sexual relations outside marriage were found in studies during the 1930s through the 1960s (Burgess & Wallin, 1953; Ehrmann, 1959; Kinsey et al., 1953; Reiss, 1967; Terman, 1938). Men tended to think that sexual intimacy was acceptable in love as well as casual relationships, while women thought that sex outside a love relationship was unacceptable. Attitudinal differences between the sexes began to wane in the mid 1960s and continued to decline through the 1970s (Croake & James, 1973; DeLameter & MacCorquodale, 1979; Hunt, 1974; Packard, 1968; Reiss, 1976; Sorensen, 1973; Yankelovich, 1974).

Also occurring during this time were attitude changes toward petting and sexual intercourse among high school and college students, with the greatest changes occurring in female attitudes toward permissiveness (Bell & Chaskes, 1970; Christensen & Gregg, 1970; Ferrell, Tolone, & Walsh, 1977; Glenn & Weaver, 1979; Robinson, King, & Balsivick, 1972; Yankelovich, 1974; Zelnik & Kantner, 1977). By far the greatest shifts in attitude have occurred among high school, rather than college, graduates. In comparison with young girls in the 1970s, today's adolescents seem to move on to intercourse rather than limit themselves to heavy petting. The greater availability of contraceptive methods, as well as increasingly liberal attitudes toward nonmarital coitus, may account for this (Chilman, 1986).

There are regional differences in sexual attitudes, with Southerners being the most conservative and Eastern and Western inhabitants of the United States being the most liberal. Black males tend to be more permissive than any other group studied, and black females are more lenient in their attitudes toward nonmarital sex than are white females (Reiss, 1967; Yankelovich, 1974).

Of interest is the fact that liberal attitudes toward sexual relations are associated with sexual experience. This has been found to be especially true among white females and males and slightly less so among blacks. It is impossible to ascertain, however, whether liberal attitudes precede sexual experience or vice versa. Many white girls, for example, claim to have agreed to sex, not because they approved of intercourse for themselves but because their boyfriends expected it of them (Cvetkovich & Grote, 1976).

A thorough understanding of changing attitudes toward sexuality can be understood only in light of the social, political, and economic variables of particular time periods. For instance, increasingly permissive attitudes toward sexual behavior, especially among females, accompanied other societal changes such as greater acceptance of cohabitation, open marriage, and divorce. Similarly, the legalization of abortion, sex education in the schools, legislation prohibiting the exclusion of pregnant girls from regular public education, and the availability of contraceptives to minors were significant events affecting adolescent sexuality. Changes in public opinion toward more positive attitudes regarding unwed motherhood; the feminist movement; increased occurrence of divorce, separation, and remarriage; inflation and the entry of more mothers into the job force (75% of the mothers of teens); the growing feminization of poverty; and the high rate of youth unemployment are also factors related to increased permissiveness and rising rates of intercourse among teens (Chilman, 1986).

Chilman argues that divorce is a highly disruptive event that often deprives the adolescent of needed stability during a vulnerable stage of development. If their parents remarry, many adolescents have the difficult task of adjusting to new and complex relationships with stepparents and stepsiblings (Chilman, 1983). The increasing number of working mothers affords teens unsupervised time and a place for coitus. Zelnick and Kantner, in their 1980 study, found that adolescent intercourse is most likely to occur in the teenager's own home while parents are at work. They also cite the greater incidence of premarital sex among teens who come from one-parent, low-income families. It seems that adolescents from such environments often experience deprivations in affection, security, and a sense of significance, which lead them to seek fulfillment elsewhere.

From an economic point of view, youth unemployment and the availability of Aid for Families with Dependent Children (AFDC) benefits, may be related to sexual promiscuity. Youth who perceive that graduating from high school is no guarantee of employment often lack motivation in their educational or vocational pursuits. In this case the argument against unprotected sexual behavior because of its negative impact on one's future economic status loses credence. The AFDC issue relates to the question of whether the availability of welfare funds encourages sexual behavior and childbirth outside marriage. According to research by Ross and Sawhill (1975) and Moore and Caldwell (1977), this is not the case. Rather it increases a teen's options and allows her more freedom of choice as to pregnancy outcome and her marital status.

A final consideration in an overview of changing mores is the social unrest of the Vietnam era. From the late 1960s to the early 1970s, social criticism, increasing alienation, and questioning of traditional social values were prevalent. Students polled regarding social attitudes in 1969 and again in 1973 strongly favored more sexual freedom. However, by the late 1970s there was evidence that American youth were turning toward more conservative sexual attitudes (Robinson & Jedlicka, 1982; Singh, 1980). With rising health concerns in the 1980s regarding the transmission of AIDS, it is possible that adolescent sexuality will once again be affected by the social and political climate of the nation.

Puberty and Maturation

Though data in this area are scanty, there may be a relationship between biological maturity and sexual attitudes and experimentation. Early studies from 1948 and 1963 found that early-maturing boys were likely to engage in sexual activities earlier than late-maturing boys. Though a similar pattern was found for girls, it was not as strong (Chilman, 1963; Kinsey et al., 1948).

Rogel and his associates studied sexuality in black females and found a relationship between timing of menarche and sexual attitudes and behavior. In his sample girls who had experienced earlier onset of menses reported having more positive attitudes toward sex. This did not predict earlier experiences of first intercourse and pregnancy for these girls, however. The early-maturing females delayed both events longer than "on-time" females, with the result that both groups had similar age equivalents for these experiences (Rogel, Fleming, & Zuehlke, 1981).

A controversial study by Udry (1983) revealed a strong relationship for males and females of both races between maturational age and sexual relations. In Presser's 1978 study, however, age and maturity were related to sexual activity for black girls only. Because of the contradictory nature of findings in this area, further research is recommended (Hamburg, 1986).

Religion

Religion also plays a role in sexual promiscuity, particularly as it relates to conservative attitudes among whites. Since the 1960s the emergence of new forms of religion and increases in religiosity among a large number of young people may have increased sexual conservatism in these groups (Chilman, 1986). In addition, a study at a southeastern university compared 1975 responses from undergraduates with 1980 responses and found that a higher number of students in 1980 reported nonmarital sex as immoral. Nonetheless, in the 1980 study the actual rate of sexual intercourse among the students was higher than reported in the 1965 study (Robinson & Jedlicka, 1982).

Education

Education interacts with other variables to affect a teen's likelihood of engaging in sexual intercourse at a young age. This is particularly true for females; having positive attitudes toward education, higher levels of achievement, and clear educational goals lessens the tendency for girls to participate in premarital sex (Gebhard, Pomeroy, Martin, & Christensen, 1956; Jessor & Jessor, 1975; Udry, Bauman, & Morris, 1975; Zelnik &

Kantner, 1980). This too is confounded, however, by various socioeconomic, psychosocial, and situational variables (higher socioeconomic status, work vs. play orientation, higher levels of cognitive development, ability to plan for the future, etc.), which may also play a role in deterring young girls from sexual activity.

Psychological Variables

Cvetkovich and Grote (1976) studied sexually active adolescents and found that sexually experienced males exhibited more risk-taking and permissive attitudes toward sexual relations than their virgin counterparts, and fewer thought of themselves as religious. For females, sexual activity appeared significantly tied to traditional female sex roles, with many girls indicating they participated in intercourse because their boyfriends expected it.

Sexually active young teens were found by Jessor and Jessor (1975) to have lower grade point averages in school, lower achievement expectations, and less acceptance of parental controls. Additionally, they tended to place independence and deviance in a more positive light than did virgins of both sexes, maintained more permissive attitudes toward sex, regarded their parents as more accepting of deviance, and generally felt more accepted by peers. Though sexually active adolescent males were found to have higher self-esteem ratings than did virgin males, this was not the case for girls.

Nonvirgin girls tended to place a higher value on affection and were likely to feel they received little support from their parents. These girls also viewed their parents as being in conflict with their friends, were more socially critical and alienated, and deemed themselves less religious than did virgin girls.

Socioeconomic Status

Lower socioeconomic status of a teen's family has been linked with early age of intercourse among females, particularly among blacks (Zelnick, Kantner, & Ford, 1982). A number of studies have shown that the vast majority of inner-city teens from low-income families have engaged in premarital sex (Furstenberg, 1976; Ladner 1971; Rainwater, 1970; Staples, 1973; Zelnik & Kantner, 1980). However, a study by Zelnick and Kantner (1977) revealed similar rates of nonmarital intercourse among blacks with college-educated fathers and whites of similar status.

Teens from white working-class families also tend to have higher rates of premarital intercourse. This group is more likely than blacks, however, to marry at a young age, often when unplanned pregnancies occur (Rubin, 1976). A look at other variables associated with socioeconomic status may explain the high rates of sexual promiscuity among both of these groups. For urban blacks, adverse conditions associated with poverty, poor educational facilities, high unemployment, fatalistic attitudes, and the need to "prove" oneself may play a significant role in early sexual experimentation (Chilman, 1986; Kessler & Cleary, 1980). Rubin found similar attitudes among whites from blue-collar families, who felt they had little to look forward to in life and no real reason to plan for the future.

Family Relations

There appears to be a link between parent-youth relationships and adolescent sexual behavior. Adolescents who have mothers with nontraditional attitudes are more likely to engage in premarital relations than those teens coming from more traditional families. This is particularly so when the mothers have difficulty combining mild, firm discipline with affection toward their children. Additionally, rates of teen intercourse are higher for adolescents from single-parent families, for those who are unhappy at home, and for those who feel they have poor communication with their parents (DeLameter & MacCorquodale, 1979; Fox, 1979; Jessor & Jessor, 1975; Kantner & Zelnick, 1972; Ladner, 1971; Reiss, 1967; Sorensen, 1973; Zelnik et al., 1982).

Effects of Drugs and Alcohol

The use and abuse of drugs and alcohol appear to be higher among teens participating in premarital sex than among their virgin counterparts (Jessor & Jessor, 1975). Though teens who engage in these activities typically have lowered inhibitions, possibly resulting in higher rates of sexual experimentation and unprotected intercourse, it is unclear whether liberal attitudes toward adolescent sexuality are a result of drug and alcohol use or whether these teens tend to have more liberal attitudes in general. Other studies have shown a link between sexual activity and the use of hard drugs only (Arafat & Yorburg, 1973; Vener & Stewart, 1974).

Sexual Knowledge

Adolescents' knowledge about sexuality and reproduction increases throughout the teen years (Reichelt & Werley, 1975; Zelnick & Kantner, 1979). Approximately 62% of American females have had a sex education class in a school setting by the age of 15. Unfortunately, exposure to sex education does not guarantee that an adolescent will have gained adequate knowledge about sexual matters. A possible explanation for this is that educational techniques may not be targeting cognitive levels of certain adolescent subgroups and that the content may not be relevant to their stage of development. Additionally, the material disseminated may be too didactic in nature and of little practical use to teenagers. Unfortunately, parental resistance to sex education in some school districts has been instrumental in keeping sexual matters from being discussed in that setting at all (Hamburg, 1986).

With such scanty information available to teens in school, one would hope for high levels of communication about sexuality at home. This is not the case, however, and studies have repeatedly shown that adolescents never cite their parents as a major source of information about sex (Bloch, 1972; Fox, 1979; Rothenberg, 1978). Nonetheless, the impact of parental communication about sexuality has been found to be significant, resulting in postponement of age of initial sexual activity. In families with females who are already sexually active, discussions about sex appear to be related to more effective use of birth control methods (Fox, 1979; Furstenberg, 1976).

Though physicians are viewed by adolescents as potentially good sources of information, teenagers rarely visit them. Thus, most teens must depend on often faulty or distorted information gleaned from the media or their peers to guide them in sexual matters (Yankelovich, Skelly, & White, Inc., 1979).

Peers are known to play a role in the permissive adolescent's life, and males appear to be most strongly influenced by their peer group's sexual behavior. Again, it is unclear whether teens choose friends whose beliefs are compatible with their own or if they conform to the sexual attitudes of their friends (Chilman, 1979; Scales & Beckstein, 1982).

TEEN CONTRACEPTIVE BEHAVIORS

"I wasn't using birth control. I thought about it sometimes, but I figured if I got pregnant, I got pregnant."

"I was at a party and had too much to drink. I never planned to have sex, and never dreamed I would become pregnant."

"My boyfriend told me I wouldn't get pregnant because he would withdraw. I believed him."

"I didn't want it to be like I *planned* to have sex."

"I just never thought it would happen to me."

These are statements frequently heard from teens who did not plan their pregnancies. In some cases adolescents are ambivalent about the possibility of becoming pregnant, and their birth control practices reflect this. In most cases, however, teens either are poorly informed about adequate protective measures or use contraceptive methods ineffectively.

Consistent use of effective methods of birth control increases with the adolescent's age. As mentioned previously, 1 out of 3 teenagers does not use any contraception the first time she has intercourse. Most wait about a year after becoming sexually active before seeking contraceptives (Furstenberg, 1981; Zabin & Clark, 1981). Early adolescents are notoriously poor contraceptors. Results from 1976 indicate that nearly 40% of sexually active 15-year-olds had never used contraception, and only 30% consistently used any method of contraception (Zelnick & Kantner, 1977). For those teens motivated enough to seek contraceptive devices, among 14-year-olds only half then used them, and for 15-year-olds only two thirds were consistent users (Akpom, Akpom, & Davis, 1976).

Studies have shown that 30% of sexually active teens use a medical or drugstore method (pill, IUD, diaphragm, foam, condoms, or suppositories); however, only 25% are regular users. This leaves more than 3.5 million teenagers at risk for pregnancy (Planned Parenthood, 1985).

Though teens as a group have increased their use of contraceptives during the past few years, pregnancy rates have also increased. The reasons for this are possibly twofold: (1) a shift away from the most effective contraceptive measures (i.e., oral contraceptives and the IUD) and (2) adolescents becoming sexually active at increasingly younger ages, thus lengthening the risk period in which teens are likely to have unprotected intercourse (Zelnik et al., 1981).

Many sexually active young girls depend on male methods of contraception. Unfortunately, adolescent males are highly inconsistent in their use of contraception, possibly lacking concern about pregnancy prevention, thus greatly increasing the risk of pregnancy for teens relying on male means of protection (Brown, Lieberman, & Miller, 1975; Finkel & Finkel, 1975; Sorensen, 1973; Zelnik & Kantner, 1980). Black males appear to be particularly lax in their use of contraception (Cvetkovich & Grote, 1976; Finkel & Finkel, 1975).

Lindemann (1974) has suggested a three-stage model of contraception that he feels characterizes the developmental aspects of adolescent sexuality. His first stage, the *natural* stage, is characterized by recent involvement in heterosexual relationships; little, if any, awareness of the need for contraception or the possibility of pregnancy; sporadic, unpredictable coitus; and a belief in the spontaneity of sex.

Stage 2 is the *peer prescription* stage. In this phase teens seek out friends for information about sexuality and experiment with nonprescription methods of birth control. A major problem in this stage is misinformation.

In the *expert* stage, adolescents exhibit a willingness to seek professional aid in obtaining a prescribed method of contraception. Adolescents in this stage are likely to be involved in a steady relationship, be committed to and have intercourse more frequently, and be more developmentally mature.

Demographic, situational, and psychological variables have been found to be associated with the failure of adolescents to use effective means of contraception (Cvetkovich & Grote, 1976; DeLameter & MacCorquodale, 1979; Finkel & Finkel, 1975; Flaherty, Maracek, Olsen, & Wilcove, 1982; Fox & Inazu, 1980; Furstenberg, 1976, 1980; Goldsmith, Gabrielson, & Gabrielson, 1972; Hornick, Doran, & Crawford, 1979; Jorgenson, King, & Torrey, 1980; Ladner, 1971; Lindemann, 1974; Luker, 1975; Miller, 1976; Mindick & Oskamp, 1982; Moyer & de Rosenroll, 1984; Presser, 1977; Rogel, Zuehlke, Petersen, Tobin-Richards, & Shelton, 1980; Rosen, Martindale, & Grisdela, 1976; Shah, Zelnik, & Kantner, 1975; Zelnik & Kantner, 1977, 1980; Zelnik, Kantner, & Ford, 1982).

Demographic variables linked with lack of, or ineffective use of, contraception include age younger than 18, nonmarital and lower socioeconomic status, membership in a minority group, fundamentalist religious affiliation, and nonenrollment in college.

Situational variables that have been reported are lack of a steady committed relationship; sporadic, unplanned intercourse; unavailability of contraceptives at the time of need; never having experienced a pregnancy; high-stress situation; unavailability of free, confidential family planning services not requiring parental consent; and poor communication with parents regarding contraceptives.

Among psychological variables cited are lack of awareness of pregnancy risks and family planning services; wanting a baby or high fertility values; traditional female attitudes and/or passivity and dependency; feelings of powerlessness, fatalism, alienation, or trusting to luck; lack of future goals and low educational achievement; high anxiety and low self-esteem; denial of sexual behavior or that pregnancy can occur; poor relationship with parents; poor communication about sex and contraceptives between parents and youth and among couples; chaotic family situation; lack of awareness of parents' experience with contraceptives; risk- and pleasure-seeking attitudes; fear of infertility or side effects or the experience of physical side effects due to contraceptives; misconceptions regarding the "safe time" of the menstrual cycle; poor problem-solving skills or inability to plan effectively; immature level of cognition; and peer group attitudes and experiences. Finally, having friends and siblings who have become adolescent parents increases the likelihood that sexually active teens will be poor contraceptors.

Given this web of often interrelated variables, it is clear that no single factor or group of factors can adequately predict adolescent contraceptive behaviors. The relative importance of any one of these factors varies across populations, and even in seemingly identical populations the results are inconsistent. Thus, Rogel and Zuehlke (1982) call for the study of specified subgroups of adolescents, which they believe will yield more information than has previously been gained by studying sexually active adolescents as a homogeneous group.

The availability of family planning services to adolescents was made possible by federal funding in the 1970s. A substantial number of teenagers obtain contraceptive devices from such clinics each year, and an estimated 367,000 unwanted pregnancies were prevented in 1981 through these services (Torres, Forrest, & Eisman, 1981). Unfortunately, having access to contraceptives does not ensure their effective use; thus, a search for ways to enhance proper use of contraception among adolescents has been launched. A promising area has been increasing communication among adolescents and their parents. (A comprehensive review of strategies for preventing teenage pregnancy is presented in chapter 6.)

WHEN TEENS BECOME PREGNANT *reactions from friends + family*

I was surprised, and I guess I was really scared. I knew my mom would be really disappointed in me. My boyfriend was really excited though. Some of our friends have kids and he thought it was neat that he'd have one too. I didn't tell my mom for a long time. When I did she cried, but she got over it, and then she was kind of excited too. Of course there was no question that I would keep it. I don't believe in abortion.

When my boyfriend and I had sex I thought we were pretty careful about the right time of the month and stuff. I just couldn't believe I was pregnant. I figured my parents would kill me if they found out—they just wouldn't understand. My boyfriend and I decided that abortion was the only solution. I was really depressed, but I still feel like I did the right thing.

When I got pregnant at 16 it was just the worst thing. I really just didn't know what to do. I thought about abortion, but I don't think it's right. I knew I couldn't keep the baby, so I figured adoption might be a good thing. I looked into an agency and found out how many people were wanting to adopt newborn babies. It made me feel good to think that I would be able to make somebody happy by giving them my baby. It wasn't as easy as I thought though; it was really hard to give the baby up when it was time. But I kept reminding myself how much better off she would be with them and what a better life she would have. I still think about her all the time.

The result of increasingly younger adolescents becoming involved in nonmarital coitus is frequently unplanned, often unwanted, pregnancies. When adolescents become pregnant there are no easy answers. Basically three options await them: abortion, carrying the baby to term and placing it for adoption, or keeping the baby. Robertson (1981) believes this constitutes a time of "acute psychological stress" for the pregnant teenager, regardless of the outcome she considers.

A select subgroup of teenagers desire to have babies at an early age, and to them the news of confirmed pregnancy is met with joy. For others, denial of sexual activity or the ability to conceive renders them disbelieving when confronted with an unwanted pregnancy. Some continue in denial, refusing to face the reality of the pregnancy itself. Often by the time they accept the truth, a routine abortion procedure cannot be performed due to the advanced age of the fetus, and they find their options are reduced.

The Decision-Making Process

Most recent studies show that adoption is rarely seriously considered by adolescents. Instead, most opt for early abortion or carrying the pregnancy to term, planning to raise the baby themselves. Interest in how women make these difficult decisions has spurred some research in the area. To date, there is no evidence that teens choosing delivery differ from those choosing abortion when compared on issues of sex-role identity; self-esteem; or such emotional factors as anxiety, depression, or hostility (Carlson, Kaiser, Yeaworth, & Carlson, 1984; Center for Population Research, 1983; Guttentag, Salasin, & Belle, 1980).

An interesting study by Bracken, Klerman, and Bracken (1978) examined the decision-making process in pregnant, never-married black adolescents to determine what factors regulate women's choice of pregnancy outcome. Though the mean age of their sample was 20 years old, information gleaned from this study is deemed appropriate to the study of adolescent decision-making in pregnancy. In particular, Bracken et al. found that circumstances surrounding the conception, the girl's reaction to the pregnancy, communication with significant others, previous pregnancies, and availability of role models greatly influenced the decision to deliver or abort.

In general, the women in this study responded to the news of their pregnancies with sadness, anxiety, and the pervasive feeling that the pregnancy was ill timed. This is not to say, however, that the pregnancies were totally unexpected; quite the opposite was true. Although women choosing to deliver their babies were somewhat more anxious, they tended to be happier about the pregnancy and were less likely to feel it was a bad time to be pregnant. Half of the women choosing delivery had determined their choice prior to discovering they were pregnant. This compares to less than a quarter of the aborting group, although most of the women in this group made their decision to abort within 1 month of suspecting they were pregnant.

Most women choosing abortion had used a method of contraception that required the cooperation of their partner. Discussion and agreement about use of contraceptives were low in both delivering and aborting groups; however, women choosing abortion were more likely than those delivering to have talked with their partners about contraceptives.

Aborting females were twice as likely as those delivering to have sisters who had experienced an abortion; over half had at least one friend who had had an abortion. Both groups sought out their partners and/or best girlfriends when making their decisions. For women choosing delivery, their mothers were twice as likely to be involved. Sources of support for women choosing abortion were their physician and best girlfriend (in that order) and, for those delivering, their best girlfriend and partner. For those aborting there was significantly less discussion of the decision with others and, consequently, far less support for their decision.

Number and outcome of previous pregnancies appear to be related to the decision-making process of unplanned pregnancy. Women pregnant for the first time who chose abortion tended to have known their partner for less than a year. Additionally, those aborting, no matter what their previous pregnancy status, were three times as likely as those delivering to have used contraception that required the partner's cooperation.

Repression was noted among aborting females who had experienced previous abortions as well as those choosing abortion as a solution to their first pregnancy. Nonetheless, the most positive attitudes toward abortion were found in women aborting their first pregnancies.

Expected guilt was higher among women who had had previous abortions and were aborting again than for those anticipating their first abortion. For women who had delivered all previous pregnancies, those aborting the current pregnancy felt they were receiving less support for their decision than any other group. Conversely, women delivering their current pregnancies after having delivered all previous pregnancies were likely to feel they were receiving more support than any other group.

Women who had been involved with their partners over a longer period of time were more likely to choose delivery over abortion. Most of the women choosing delivery had been having sexual relations with their boyfriend for over a year. Of interest is the fact that these females were the least likely to have been using contraception, despite their lengthy sexual relationships. Those choosing to deliver their first pregnancy were the least likely to have used contraception. Additionally, women who had previously delivered another child were happier but more anxious than other groups.

Delivering females in this study perceived they had more support for their decisions than their counterparts who chose to abort, regardless of the number of previous pregnancies. Furthermore, for women opting to deliver, single-parent role models were found to be especially important determinants. Not only did women choosing to deliver know more single parents than did women aborting, but they also perceived them as receiving more support than did the aborting group. Finally, women planning to deliver did not appear worried about changes in their life-style afterwards.

Though Bracken et al. caution that the findings from their study are not generalizable to all groups of women, their data shed much light on the decision-making processes of unmarried, lower-income, primarily black females. Before concluding, however, it should be noted that half of the women in the aborting group had delivered at least one child in the past. Similarly, half of those currently delivering had experienced at least one abortion. Thus, these researchers suggest that it is not an inherent personality characteristic of the woman that will predict the outcome she will choose for any given pregnancy, but rather the unique circumstances surrounding each pregnancy.

The Decision to Abort

The choice of abortion appears to be closely tied to the socioeconomic status of the pregnant female. Those girls whose families remain intact and whose parents have higher incomes, education levels, or occupational status are most likely to choose abortion. Additionally, these girls are typically more academically motivated, are doing better in school, and are described in general as more independent, motivated, and optimistic about their futures (Chesler & Davis, 1980; Klerman, Bracken, Jekel, & Bracken, 1982; Olson, 1980).

There is some evidence to suggest that adolescents who choose abortion are likely to have achieved some financial independence from their parents and are less likely than girls choosing to deliver to be influenced by their mothers in the decision-making process (Olson, 1980). Lewis (1980) found that aborting adolescents tended to perceive their decision as externally derived. This characteristic is developmentally consistent with adolescents' difficulty in accepting responsibility for their own behavior; nonetheless Lewis suggests that there may be some truth to the assertion that teens feel pressed into an abortion decision by family members.

Adolescents account for almost one third of all aborting women (Klerman, 1981). Among countries where abortion is reported by age of mother, the United States had the highest percentage of reported legal abortions for teens in 1976 (Centers for Disease Control, 1978). With what information is available, it appears that approximately 40% of all teenage conceptions result in spontaneous or induced abortion (Robertson, 1981).

The number of abortions performed each year since legalization of abortion in 1973 has risen steadily. In 1977 over 300,000 legal abortions were performed on teenagers. A breakdown by age group reveals the largest number of abortions were performed on girls 18 to 19 years of age (189,000), the second on girls 15 to 17 years old (135,000), and the third on girls 14 and under (13,000). For these age groups only the 14-and-under group had more abortions than live births (1,132 abortions per 1,000 live births). Until recently, abortion seemed to be more acceptable to white females than to blacks. However, data from 1973 to 1977 showed a marked increase in abortions among blacks (Forrest, Sullivan, & Tietze, 1979).

Many women weigh the decision to abort against the medical, social, and psychological risks of bearing and raising a child at an early age: early curtailment of education, unemployment or low-paying jobs, frequent dependence on public assistance, and high rates of divorce. Such factors tend to have a negative impact on children of adolescents, affecting the children's emotional, social, and cognitive development and ultimately their school achievement. This is the case despite increases in the quality and the availability of prenatal care, which lessens the risk of biological damage to the developing fetus (Baldwin & Cain, 1980). Nonetheless it is important for girls choosing abortion to understand the risks involved in that decision. From a medical standpoint the risks of abortion are minimal. During 1977 only 15 deaths (1.4 per 100,000 abortions) were reported. The medical risks are therefore less than that of a young girl choosing childbirth or undergoing a routine tonsillectomy.

The risk of abortion has declined over the past few years and appears related to the fact that females are presenting for abortion during earlier phases of pregnancy. During the period from 1972 to 1976, death rates for legal abortion were lowest for women seeking abortions at less than 8 weeks gestational age. For gestational ages between 9 and 10 weeks, the risk to the mother was three times as great, and for abortions performed after 21 weeks, the death ratio was nearly 45 times as great as for those under 8 weeks (Robertson, 1981).

Complications of abortion are also related to gestational age at presentation. Robertson cites perforation of the uterus, severe pelvic infection, and cervical injury as possible negative outcomes of abortion. In extreme cases, major abdominal surgery is mandated. All of the above may have profound effects on a woman's future pregnancies. Though research on the impact of abortion on future pregnancies has produced conflicting results, two fairly recent studies have suggested that abortion does not significantly increase a female's risk of miscarriage, prematurity, or other negative outcomes (e.g., Harlap, Shiono, Ramcharan, et al., 1979; Institute of Medicine, 1975).

There was some initial concern that legalization of abortion would result in exploitation of abortion as a form of birth control. Because multiple abortions are viewed as an increased risk to future pregnancies, and because federal funds were involved, investigators sought to confirm the dread hypothesis. An early study performed in New York City revealed that the availability of legal abortion had not led to exploitation but rather to more effective means of pregnancy prevention (Tietze, 1975).

Similarly, Evans, Selstad, and Welcher (1976) studied a group of teens whose first pregnancies had been terminated by abortion. For these girls

4 out of 5 reported consistent use of an effective method of birth control after the abortion. This was equivalent to the rates of those who had delivered their babies and higher than the rates of effective use by girls who had never experienced a pregnancy. In his 1976 study Darney found that postabortion adolescents were more accepting of birth control methods on hospital discharge than were teens who had delivered. This was the case for all groups (both black and white), except teens 14 and under.

The social and economic consequences of bearing a child often come into play in an adolescent's decision to abort. For many the transient discomforts associated with an abortion are far more favorable than the short- and long-term consequences of teenage motherhood and parenting. Though feelings of regret, guilt, or loss may be experienced following abortion, these are usually only temporary and appear to be counterbalanced by more prevalent feelings of relief and "positive life changes" (Institute of Medicine, 1975). Perez-Reyes and Falk (1973) found that 75% of 13- to 16-year-olds experienced the same or better levels of emotional health 6 months after the procedure. The same was true for the physical health of the aborting teens, as 90% reported that their physical health was the same or better after the abortion.

Of interest in the Perez-Reyes and Falk study was the use of the Minnesota Multiphasic Personality Inventory (MMPI) to measure personality changes in the adolescents as a result of abortion. The results indicated that adolescents considering abortion are likely to be confused, sad, suspicious of others, sensitive, and worried, having many physical concerns and feeling poorly about themselves. Retesting these individuals 6 months after their abortions, it appeared that for early adolescents abortion relieved stress rather than exacerbating it. However, the study did not compare the relief of teens choosing abortion with those choosing delivery, and it is uncertain whether gains in positive mental health are unique to girls who abort or whether girls who have delivered their babies have similar positive outcomes (Klerman et al., 1982). Graves (1976) compared both aborting and delivering teens and concluded that legal abortions were no more likely to cause psychological distress than carrying a baby to term.

An interesting California study of Mexican-American and Anglo-Saxon 13- to 19-year-olds compared pre- and postattitudes of delivering and aborting pregnant girls. Posttesting done 6 months after abortion or delivery of the infant revealed that teens became more satisfied with whatever decision they had made over time. Many of the aborting teens who had indicated abortion was not their first choice had come to see that it had indeed been the best choice for them. Twenty percent of this group, however, expressed regret over their decision to abort. The researchers were later able to identify the unhappy individuals on the basis of their pretests, in that these females initially exhibited greater ambivalence about their decisions, were younger, came from a minority group, and had poorer educational backgrounds.

Females who choose abortion with the support of their spouse, significant other, or mothers (for unmarried teens) are more likely to have positive reactions to their abortions. Women for whom the decision to abort is very difficult appear more prone to postabortion guilt and anxiety (Bracken et al., 1978). In summary, abortion responses from teenagers are similar to those of older women: possible transient depression following the procedure, but no long-term or permanent psychological impairment as a result of the abortion.

The reaction of males to the news of unwanted pregnancy varies; however, when abortion is the chosen outcome, males are often reportedly upset, confused, and worried, frequently complaining that they have been excluded from the decision-making process (Wade, 1977). Additionally, some men express concern that they have no legal rights concerning their girlfriend's (or wife's) decision to terminate the pregnancy (Collier, 1980).

In conclusion, attitudes toward abortion appear to be affected by events surrounding conception and the decision-making process involved in unplanned pregnancy. Nearly all women experience a great deal of stress and conflict over their decision to abort. For some the ethical aspects of abortion weigh heavily in their decision not to abort. However, it should be noted that attitudes toward abortion appear to change with one's experience of it (Bracken et al., 1978). Thus, when seeking to predict pregnancy outcome choices, the circumstances of each individual pregnancy should be reviewed, rather than relying on underlying personality characteristics or attitudes of the pregnant adolescent.

Adoption

Adoption, the traditional solution to the problem of unwanted pregnancies, is no longer in vogue and is rarely considered by today's youth. In study after study, teens report that adoption was never an option they considered (e.g., Bracken et al., 1978; Klerman et al., 1982). For the most part teens indicate that they do not want to carry the pregnancy to term if they are not going to keep the infant. Though prolife advocates encourage girls to relinquish their infants, only about 10% do (Chilman, 1979; Klerman, 1981; Klerman et al., 1982).

When adolescents choose adoption, there are often many periods of vacillation and indecision throughout the pregnancy and following delivery. Even the most adamant can change her mind; thus, laws protect the relinquishing mother for a given period, usually 90 days after the birth, wherein she can decide to keep the child. Teens who give up their babies may experience feelings of loss or guilt over abandonment of the child as well as recurrent sadness on the child's birthdays (Authier & Authier, 1982).

For childless couples seeking to adopt, the current situation is indeed bleak. With more and more adolescents choosing abortion or opting to raise their babies themselves, few babies become available for adoption. One recent estimate is that for every white baby available for adoption there are 60 families hoping to adopt it (Quinlen, 1987). Along with the decreasing availability of newborns, infertility rates appear to be on the rise as a result of delayed childbirth among many career women and more widespread venereal disease.

Parents seeking to adopt are typically 25- to 35-year-old suburbanites who are active churchgoers with annual incomes averaging $25,000. A large number of these childless couples have been trying to conceive for many years. At present, there are an estimated 3 million such couples hoping to adopt (Quinlen, 1987). Those seeking the services of adoption agencies have faced waiting lists 2 or 3 years long. Recently, many agencies have stopped taking applications, and some have closed their doors altogether. There simply are not enough babies available to keep the agencies functioning.

In desperation, some would-be parents advertise nationwide, offering to pay a pregnant girl's medical and living expenses until the baby is born. Others contact physicians in the hope that their name will be given to unwed mothers wanting to relinquish their babies at birth. As babies become harder to come by, increasing numbers of American couples look to foreign countries to adopt unwanted or homeless children.

Private or independent adoption, though not legal in every state, has become more prevalent in the past few years as agencies have failed to meet the increasing demand for infants. In all cases the law mandates that the biological parents formally relinquish their legal rights to the child. When the baby is illegitimate, only the mother's consent is required, although there are various stipulations about notifying the father. Strict laws in every state prohibit the sale of babies, allowing the mother to receive compensation only for medical and living expenses during her pregnancy.

The increasing trend toward private adoptions is often criticized by child welfare authorities who claim there is too little screening of the prospective parents' ability to successfully care for and raise a child. In extreme cases the only requirements the adopting couple must meet are the desire for a child and the ability to meet adoption expenses. The emotional needs of the biological mother are frequently neglected in such transactions. Additionally, medical histories of the natural parents, which could have a profound effect on the infant, are too often not provided to the adopting couple, thus placing all parties at a disadvantage (Greer, 1982).

Childless couples have come to see some states as preferable to others when seeking a private adoption. In Charleston, South Carolina, for example, lax laws allow out-of-state couples to adopt privately through local court proceedings. Critics of the process fear that couples rejected by licensed agencies in other states are permitted to adopt through South Carolina's system, where waiver of strict home studies is common. They also claim that offering sometimes confused and vulnerable pregnant adolescents large sums of money (frequently surpassing their actual medical and living expenses) encourages girls to surrender their infants too readily, a decision they may later regret. Additionally, child-hungry couples with available resources may spawn undesirable "shopping" on the part of teens, who may go looking for the highest bidder.

A new concept in adoption called *open adoption* may make it easier for girls to relinquish their babies. Here a female wishing to place her child with an adoptive family can peruse the files of hopeful couples and choose the family she would like to take custody of her child. For many teens this eases the guilt and indecision of the adoptive process in that they have an active role in choosing the kind of home and the parents the baby will have (Quinlen, 1987).

One of the many tragedies of teenage motherhood is that mothers who originally plan to blissfully raise their infants while completing school and growing up themselves often find the burdens of motherhood overwhelming. Their children frequently make their way into foster placement and may later become available for adoption. Current legislation and adoption agency staff are focusing their efforts on placing these older children. Additionally, there are increasing efforts to place emotionally impaired or physically handicapped children into childless homes. Such children number around 200,000 in the United States and constitute a group of children termed hard-to-place.

The "baby shortage" has spawned a number of other options for childless couples, one of which is surrogate motherhood. Early critics of this process claimed that surrogatism would lead to a "breeder class" of poor women bearing children for the rich. To the contrary, however, it appears that females who volunteer as surrogates are likely to be educated women from middle-class backgrounds that are very similar to those of the couples with whom they contract. The typical surrogate loves being pregnant, reporting that life is at its best while one is carrying a child. Additionally, many women indicate that unresolved feelings from an abortion or a child given up for adoption prompted them to contract as surrogates.

In sum, present trends toward teenage parenting have reached far beyond the adolescent's own home. The dearth of available infants, coupled with increasing rates of infertility as women postpone childbearing, has created a real crisis for many childless couples. Those hoping to adopt often face long years of waiting for a child, some pursue private adoptions through physicians and attorneys, and others look outside the United States for foreign adoptions. Both private adoption and surrogate motherhood have been viewed negatively by those who fear the exploitation of mother and child. Efforts are currently being directed toward encouraging hopeful couples to adopt older or minority children or children who may be emotionally or physically impaired.

Teen Parenting

Why do some adolescents choose to have babies? This is a question many experts are currently asking. Perhaps it is a sense of worthlessness and despair or feelings of lack of opportunity that lead many teens to motherhood. Some girls may feel there is simply no interesting alternative to childrearing. It is speculated that teenagers with a history of deprivation or neglect may view mothering as a means of getting their nurturing and security needs met. In some cases having a baby may be a legitimate attempt to grow up, and some adolescents may view mothering as the only route to economic independence. Early parenting and marriage allow many females to strengthen their identities with their mothers, while establishing their own feminine role and identity. Further, early marriage may provide adolescents with a socially acceptable way to gratify their increasing sexual desires (Buchholz & Gol, 1986).

Early work in the area led Komarovsky (1962) to view teenage motherhood as following a family or class pattern. Most, he observed, had fathers (and often husbands) belonging to the working class. In many cases the adolescents had mothers, sisters, and girlfriends who married while teens. Neither they nor their parents held expectations for higher education or career training; thus, most dropped out of school between the seventh and eleventh grades. Komarovsky viewed marriage as the "career of choice" for these girls and indicated that they did not appear to face the same conflict over choosing between marriage and college or a career as girls from higher socioeconomic backgrounds. As a cultural component, Labarre (1968) adds that at that time many from the working class considered 14- to 16-year-olds mature enough for marriage and motherhood.

Whatever the motivation for youthful childbearing, the consequences of teen parenting are long term—deeply affecting both mother and child and ultimately society as a whole. Teen mothers and their children are far more likely than other women with children to live in poverty. It is estimated that only half of those girls having babies before the age of 18 will complete high school. This compares with 96% of female adolescents who do not bear children during their school-age years. Largely because of early curtailment of education, teenage mothers earn approximately half as much as their nonparenting counterparts and are far more likely to receive welfare benefits. Seventy-one percent of all females under 30 presently dependent on federal assistance bore children as teenagers (Alan Guttmacher Institute, 1986).

Much research on the ill effects of teenage mothering has focused on the effects of poverty and poor medical care. However, Baldwin and Cain (1980) found that when free or low-cost medical assistance is provided to pregnant girls, the adverse effects of early childbearing on the health of the mother tend to disappear. Nonetheless, many adolescents are likely to suffer from poor nutrition, drug and alcohol experimentation and abuse, smoking, venereal disease, and anemia, all of which place them at risk before they ever become pregnant. Many of these conditions bear direct relationship to prenatal problems, serving as causal conditions for premature labor, intrauterine growth retardation, spontaneous abortion, prematurity or low birth weight, fetal death, and maternal mortality (Sacker & Neuhoff, 1982).

It should be noted that although the statistics for maternal mortality are relatively small, the rates are nearly twice as high for adolescents as for adults (e.g., Adams & Hatcher, 1977; Alan Guttmacher Institute, 1976), and the rates may increase for teens having more than one child during their teen years. For adolescents under the age of 15, mortality rates are almost 10 times those for adult women (e.g., Baldwin, 1976; Smith & Mumford, 1980).

The child of the adolescent mother faces higher rates of illness and mortality, in addition to later educational and emotional problems (Landy, Schubert, Cleland, & Montgomery, 1984). Children born to older adolescents may fare considerably better than those born to very young girls, however. A study comparing offspring of older adolescents with women in their early 20s showed no differences in early childhood health and development (Kinard & Reinherz, 1984). Additionally, it has been found that infants' health appears to be better when two adults live in the home, rather than just a single parent (Chilman, 1983). Research on attachment and bonding seems to suggest that adolescents are able to form a successful attachment to one child, but additional children stress their capabilities (Bolton, 1980). Thus, many children become innocent victims of abuse at the hands of immature, frustrated parents. Finally, for female children of adolescent parents, there is an increased risk that they too will become parents during their teen years.

There are many potential areas of stress for the new mother: The teenager may find herself cut off from peers by her family (McLanahan, Wedemeyer, & Adelberg, 1981); conflicts may arise with the grandparents over care of the infant (Cannon-Bonventre, 1979; Furstenberg, 1980); there may be strain between the mother and the child's father and their respective families (Bolton, 1980; Howard, 1979); and the pregnant/parenting adolescent may be prone to loneliness (Fine & Pape, 1982), depression (Bierman & Streett, 1982), and conflict over pregnancy outcome decisions (Bracken et al., 1978; Malmquist, Kircsuk, & Spano, 1967).

Over the years the greater acceptance of adolescent parenthood has helped eradicate many of the more obvious psychological stresses associated with early pregnancy. Nonetheless, it is apparent that teens who choose to parent find themselves subjected to demands beyond those of their nonparenting peers. In particular, it has been shown that poor or minority adolescent parents suffer emotional difficulties that last well into their children's school years (Brown, Adams, & Kellam, 1981). As Dohrenwend and Dohrenwend (1974) have pointed out, however, there is a distinct relationship between socioeconomic factors and mental health. Thus, it is possible that social and economic factors may have a greater impact on the psychological well-being of the mother than pregnancy or childrearing itself.

Traditionally, teenage mothers have been viewed as a deviant group, experiencing high levels of distress. For example, a 1970 study compiling data from 1963 to 1964 reported a high suicide rate among pregnant teenagers (Gabrielson, Klerman, Currie, Tyler, & Jekel, 1970). Several other studies from this period report similar findings of impaired mental health in this population (e.g., Sauber & Corrigan, 1970). Among traits often attributed to pregnant or parenting adolescents are low self-worth (Faigel, 1967), poor ability to make plans (Rains, 1971), risk-taking (Miller, 1973), external locus of control (Connolly, 1975; Meyerowitz & Malev, 1973), overdependence (Heiman & Levitt, 1960; Loesch & Greenberg, 1962), weak ego strength (Babikian & Goldman, 1971), self-devaluation (Kaplan, Smith, & Pokorny, 1979), anomie (Goode, 1961; Roberts, 1966), and a tendency to use denial as a defense mechanism (Rader, Bekker, Brown, & Richardt, 1978).

Other work in this area has been unsuccessful in identifying significant familial or psychological disturbances among pregnant or parenting teens (Hatcher, 1973; Meyerowitz & Malev, 1973; Pope, 1967; Ralph, Lochman, & Thomas, 1984; Vincent, 1961). Additionally, it is clear that cultural values must be considered when studying pregnant/parenting adolescents (Juhasz, 1974; McKay & Richardson, 1973). It appears, for instance, that there is more acceptance of both early pregnancy and mothering among indigent adolescents than for those from more affluent backgrounds (Goldfarb, Mumford, Shurn, Smith, Flowers, & Shum, 1977).

There has long been a search for personality or situational variables that might predict adolescent pregnancy and parenthood. Much of this

research has focused on issues of self-esteem and locus of contr\
& Allen, 1987). Abernethy, Robbins, Abernethy, Grunebaum,\
(1975) studied adolescent self-concept and found pregnant teen.   .o
have lower self-esteem than those who had never been pregnant. They
hypothesized that lower estimates of self-worth prompted these girls to
seek attention from males in ways that placed them at risk for unwanted
pregnancy. Zonger (1977) found pregnant adolescents to be more dissat-
isfied with themselves physically as well as experiencing feelings of inad-
equacy and unworthiness. It is unclear, however, whether feelings of self-
deprecation are a result of pregnancy and extreme hormonal and bodily
changes or whether pregnancy is an outcome of low feelings of self-worth.

Segal and Ducette (1973) studied perception of locus of control in
pregnant and nonpregnant teens. They found that pregnant, white middle-
class female adolescents were more likely than their nonpregnant white
classmates to report external locus of control. For black adolescent girls
the opposite was true, with pregnant teenagers scoring internal on measures
of locus of control while nonpregnant black teens scored external.

Barth, Schinke, and Maxwell (1983) found that depression was slightly
higher in pregnant groups and that self-esteem was lower for both pregnant
and parenting groups as opposed to nonpregnant, nonparenting teens.
Previous findings that adolescent pregnancy is a time of optimism and
heightened well-being (Paffenberger & McCabe, 1966) were not confirmed
by this study. Barth et al. found that for all groups circumstantial variables
predicted psychological well-being far better than did childbearing status.
An interesting finding is that both pregnant and parenting teens indicated
that they received more social support than did the control group, but the
effects of social supports were greatest for the adolescent parents.

Nelson, Gumlak, and Politano (1986) also searched for personality
differences between pregnant and nonpregnant, nonparenting adolescents
using three groups: (a) pregnant for the first time (primigravida), (b) pregnant for the second or more times (multigravida), and (c) nonpregnant,
sexually active. Using the Minnesota Multiphasic Personality Inventory
(MMPI) Nelson et al. were able to discriminate between pregnant and
nonpregnant adolescents, but they found it difficult to differentiate between
the pregnant groups. Multi- and primigravida adolescent groups reported
far more anxiety than nonpregnant teenagers. Multigravida teenagers appeared less concerned about their health and bodily functions than those
experiencing pregnancy for the first time. However, as a group, pregnant
adolescents experienced more guilt and felt more alienated, inferior, mis-
understood, and isolated. Additionally, they had more difficulty being
assertive than their nonpregnant counterparts.

Personality characteristics of both unwed mothering groups are suggestive of more chronic types of emotional difficulties, wherein the adolescents

may appear hostile, suspicious of others, irritable, tense, and anxious. In addition, conflicts regarding sexuality may be common in these groups as well as a tendency toward being narcissistic, demanding, and egocentric. Further, it appears that these pregnant teens may be prone to acting out, tending to use projection and rationalization as prominent defense mechanisms.

Conversely, the sexually active, nonpregnant adolescents exhibited characteristics of being mildly nonconforming and independent, with possible histories of minor difficulties in meeting societal demands and limitations. These individuals tended to be enthusiastic, outgoing, and sociable. However, as Nelson et al. point out, differences between pregnant and nonpregnant groups may simply be the result of the pregnancy itself. For instance, mothering teens' MMPI profiles derived from several other studies closely resembled the profiles of the nonpregnant teens in Nelson et al.'s study (Hooke & Marks, 1962; Horn, Green, Carney, & Erikson, 1975).

In sum, though many have traditionally believed that adolescents who become pregnant and bear children are driven by deep-seated emotional problems, there is little evidence to support this. Liberal attitudes toward adolescent sexuality, unwed motherhood, and single parenting have greatly eased the psychological burden of this childbearing population. Medical risks for adolescent mothers, however, remain higher than for adult women bearing children. Additionally, the offspring of adolescent parents are subject to higher rates of illness and mortality as well as educational and emotional difficulties.

Checking in on Angela a year later (see case study at beginning of chapter 1), she is optimistic. It has not been easy, but she has learned a lot. Though she thought she would never fall in love again, she realizes that time does indeed heal most wounds. She plans to be ready next time and takes the pill "just in case."

Angela is working hard to finish school, taking the baby with her each day to the alternate education facility for pregnant and parenting teens. But despite her optimism it is clear that Angela feels the strain of early parenting. When asked what counsel she would give pregnant teenagers she says emphatically, "Don't have a baby. If you do have a baby, stay in school." And that's just what she is doing.

Chapter 2

Teenage Parenting: Adaptive and Maladaptive Patterns

CASE STUDY: LaDAWN

At 3 p.m. the bell rings and 15-year-old LaDawn and her friends stroll to their school lockers to get their coats. Then they stop at the nursery to get their babies for the bus ride home.

This is an unusual day; LaDawn rarely comes to school. Her pregnancy was difficult, and some days she does not feel well. The midwestern winters are severe, too, and taking her 8-month-old son on two buses to get to school is hard, especially in bad weather. LaDawn feels tired; the baby cried all night. Maybe she'll skip school tomorrow; she's two grades behind already; the work is dull; she'll finish high school, sure—sometime. Much of the time she stays home with her mother and sister and watches the soaps. Her sister, age 16, has two children, so the babies play together. LaDawn has the emotional support of some family members and extensive child care help from her mother, grandmother, greatgrandmother, sisters,

Written in collaboration with Christine Butler.

and female friends—all of whom also have children. All financial help, however, must come from public assistance.

LaDawn still sees her baby's father. He is proud and happy about the baby's birth and was especially delighted that it's a boy, since this reflects well on his own manhood and virility. He comes to see LaDawn and the baby, and, although he does not help in child care, he does plan to spend time with his son and "teach him stuff"; he wants to make sure LaDawn and the female relatives don't make a sissy out of the boy. He says he loves LaDawn, but the couple has no plans to marry.

LaDawn says she is happy being a mother. She enjoys her child and experiences no significant problems with him, "except when he makes me mad." What then? "I don't do or say nothing to him 'cause he's just a baby. When he's bigger I guess I'll have to whop him sometimes to teach him." When should you punish children? "Oh, you know, sometimes they just gets on my nerves."

LaDawn plans to work eventually to support herself and her baby. She wants "a good job" but is vague in her notion of where and how she will obtain one. Medical, employment, and counseling services are available in her city, but LaDawn doesn't know this and doesn't have any idea of how to access anything outside her own neighborhood. It is likely that she will follow in her mother's footsteps, which has been a life of instability.

A NEW BREED OF MOTHER

Nine out of 10 teenagers who become pregnant choose to keep and raise their babies. In some cases this choice represents the lesser of evils for the girl and/or her family. In other cases the pregnancy was planned and wished for. Regardless of whether the pregnancy was desired, however, high school–age mothers vary widely in their degree of preparedness to adapt to the role of parent. Their ability to cope with the stresses of teen parenthood and their knowledge of appropriate childrearing practices directly affect the physical and mental well-being of their children. Children of adolescent mothers are at risk for a host of problems, including delayed development, academic difficulties, behavioral problems, and child abuse. The concern here is with identifying social and environmental factors that mediate or prevent these problems by enabling the adolescent to be a more effective parent.

STRESS AND SOCIAL SUPPORT

Stress is known to place individuals at increased risk for depression, anxiety, and other emotional problems. Parental stress may be experienced by a child as withdrawal of the parents' attention; imposition of added responsibility, often inappropriate to the child's age; or parental irritability, frustration, and angry outbursts. In some cases the stressors on the parents may lead to physical or psychological violence toward the child. Thus, in any family situation, factors that serve to buffer or ameliorate parental stress indirectly improve the child's situation. A large body of research supports the idea that in many situations social support provides an effective buffer against the effects of stress. Social support would thus appear to be a critical factor in helping teen mothers interact appropriately with their children. This is all the more true because adolescent mothers experience all the stressors that other single mothers face: economic pressure, difficulty in obtaining child care, overwork, and fatigue from juggling school, work, and home responsibilities. In addition, teens face added stress simply by virtue of their age: They must still undergo the emotional ups and downs of adolescence, while attempting to provide stability for a child, although they cannot yet achieve it themselves. They face social stigma, except in some minority cultures. Finally, adolescence in our culture is a training ground for adulthood only in the most general sense. Nothing in the young adolescent's experience prepares her to bear total responsibility for herself, let alone for another person. She must learn, quickly, on the job. Without adequate support, she is likely to flounder. With initial support and guidance, she may be able to cope with the transition into the adult role.

THE FAMILY: SUPPORT OR SUBSTITUTE?

The teen mother's primary source of social support usually is her family. In most cases the girl and her baby live with her parents and are at least partially supported by them until the girl is financially able to move out. In some instances the young mother may live alone or with the child's father, but the maternal grandmother remains an important source of material aid, advice, information, support, and, most often, free day care.

This arrangement has both benefits and drawbacks. Often it raises the question of who really acts as the child's parent. The maternal family may be a support for the young mother or a substitute for her. In cultural contexts in which extended families with shared childrearing duties are the norm, this may create no particular difficulty. In our culture, however, there is an assumption that childrearing and the decision-making that goes with it are entirely the responsibility of the parents. When this is not true, as in the case of some teen mothers, it may further complicate the teen's development of an adult identity.

The child of the adolescent mother may benefit from the care of a grandparent in a number of ways. If a grandfather or uncle is present in the home, some of the effects of the father's absence may be averted. Financial support is no small consideration. It often results in the child's enjoying relatively advantaged circumstances rather than poverty. This effect carries on into later years, since teen mothers who remain with their families complete more schooling than those who do not, and they attain higher occupational levels (Furstenburg & Crawford, 1978). When the teen mother is very young (under 16), grandmother care may protect the child from the effects of the mother's immaturity. Some evidence suggests (Hamburg, 1986) that regardless of education the very young teen is developmentally unready to acquire the judgment, patience, and emotional resiliency to cope with the child's behavior, offer consistent attention, or make sound choices regarding physical care. In some cases the girl's parents direct and oversee her treatment of the child and thus prevent neglect or mistreatment. As one young mother said, "I'd probably hit the kid a lot more, but my mom won't let me" (Barth & Schinke, 1984).

There is still much controversy over the effect such an arrangement has on the attachment of the infant to its mother. Might the child bond to the grandmother instead and never quite bond to the mother? Preliminary evidence (Treiman, 1986) suggests that this may not necessarily be the case. Infants may become attached to either or both maternal figures.

At issue is not the attachment of the child but the autonomy of the teen mother. The assumption of the parental role by the grandparents often produces resentment and anger in the teen. This may merely be a continuation of preexisting intergenerational conflicts. Pregnancy is often intended as a bid for adulthood, independence, and equality with the girl's mother and may be an attempt to escape from the home as a means to hurt and insult the parents. It backfires, however, by prolonging a girl's dependence on her parents, giving them still greater control, and often cutting the girl off from peers and other resources outside the family. When the girl realizes that her victory was short lived, she may vent her hostility on her baby or may vie with her mother for the child's loyalty. A tug-of-war ensues in which the baby is the loser.

Frequently, too, the assumption that grandparents provide a stable environment may be unfounded. When the teen's pregnancy is an expression of a troubled family system, there is little reason to suppose that the new infant will fare better than its mother.

THE IMPORTANCE OF EDUCATION

Obviously, the pros and cons of grandparent support vary depending on the individual situation. As a general rule, however, it appears that some support is necessary if the young mother and her child are to escape lifelong poverty. Some of the difficulties arise from the present policy in our culture of regarding adolescents as children unless they become parents, in which case they are suddenly adults. Interventions that might better prepare adolescents for the transition to adulthood could ease the conflict of roles in which many teens are enmeshed.

DEVELOPMENT OF PARENTING SKILLS

The foregoing would almost suggest that the teen mother's parenting skills, or lack thereof, are not a matter of concern as she may not be the primary caregiver. Such a conclusion would be most injudicious. Teen mothers' interactions with their babies exert a profound influence on the infants' development (Kinard & Reinherz, 1984; King & Fullard, 1982).

Interaction includes a number of maternal behaviors: physical care; rule-setting and discipline; physical and verbal contact; display of emotions, attention, and affection; and provision of toys and activities appropriate to the child's development. A major factor influencing a mother's behavior toward her child is, of course, her attitudes toward the child and toward her role as a mother. Attitudes are formed partly by cognitive expectations and ideas, partly by such emotional factors as self-esteem, depression, and perceived satisfaction with the relationship with the child.

The cognitive factor amounts, basically, to the mother's knowledge of child development and appropriate childrearing practices. Vukelich and Kliman (1985), Johnson, Loxterkamp, and Albanese (1982), and others have found that most adolescents have very inaccurate ideas of child development. They have an overall tendency to expect children's abilities to develop much earlier than is actually the case. For instance, the majority of a sample of Iowa high school students (Johnson et al., 1982) expected toddlers to walk, wash their hands, comprehend verbal instructions, and so forth, long before a child could reasonably be expected to do these things. Generally, the younger the teen the less accurate the expectations of the child. Furthermore, boys were far less accurate than girls.

IGNORANCE AS A RISK FACTOR FOR CHILD ABUSE

It seems intuitively clear that such ignorance of child development carries with it a high potential for maternal frustration, impatience, and angry blame toward the child when expectations are not met. The potential for overpunitiveness and physical abuse may be present. The Iowa study cited above yielded evidence supporting this conclusion: The high school students' ignorance of child development tended to correlate with the adoption of harsh, punitive, or abusive means of dealing with hypothetical child behavior problems. Again, boys overall showed more abusive attitudes than girls.

Johnson et al. (1982) pointed out that this sample included only non-parenting teens answering a paper-and-pencil questionnaire; a teen parent subject to the daily strains and pressures of childrearing might be even more likely to become frustrated and impatient with the child. A young mother who feels hampered by her child's dependency and harried by the demands of the child's care might be expected to want her child to "hurry and grow up." Her expectations may be even more distorted by wishful thinking than by ignorance. Impatience could also cause a young mother to be more punitive than she would appear on a questionnaire.

If teenagers are so ill informed about the needs and behavior of normal children at different ages, presumably they know much less about the needs of special children—those with medical, mental, or developmental problems. Studies indicate that teen mothers have a higher proportion of "problem" children than the general population (Simkins, 1984). It is also known that abused children are overrepresented among those with physical, intellectual, or emotional handicaps. Raising a special child is a stressful and difficult task, and those most likely to be faced with it are least equipped to cope with it. It seems likely that knowledge of child development and special children's needs, together with training in coping strategies, might buffer the stress of dealing with such a child and might give the mother a sense of increased competence. If the young mother has a sense of efficiency in being able to cope with problems as they arise, she will be less likely to lash out against the child in frustration.

KNOWLEDGE, ATTITUDES, AND BEHAVIOR

It is important to make a distinction between factual knowledge and attitude, because until recently it was assumed by many that the dissemination of knowledge about child development to teen mothers would in itself suffice to improve their parenting behaviors. This has been the premise of most of the existing teen-parent education programs. The Johnson et al. (1982) study revealed that changing the level of factual knowledge possessed by high schoolers often leaves their attitudes relatively unchanged; they may *know* proper disciplinary procedures but may see no reason to use them with any consistency. Training techniques that are effective for older parents may have to be modified for use with adolescents.

Emotional factors influence young mothers' attitudes as well as their expectations about parenthood (LaResche, Strobino, Parks, Fischer, & Smeriglio, 1981). Chapter 1 outlined affective characteristics of teen girls who become pregnant; perhaps most striking among them is lack of self-esteem, security, and goal directedness common in this population. Girls may intentionally become pregnant because they seek love, attention, and meaningful achievement; they expect the child to provide all of these things. One girl said, "I had the baby so it would love just me. This is one thing in the world that's really mine." Mothers with this sort of personal ego stake in their babies may be very nurturing and affectionate in their attitudes but also possessive and smothering (Camp & Morgan, 1984). They may pressure their children, seeking ego satisfaction through them. On the other hand, some girls who become pregnant accidentally do so because they have difficulty internalizing the fact that their actions have consequences. This is the adolescent "feeling of invulnerability"; it can result in the teen mother experiencing difficulty in taking a consistently responsible attitude toward her child's care. Finally, teen mothers are often affected by social isolation, interpersonal conflicts, and feelings of loneliness and depression, especially in the months following the baby's birth (Barth & Schinke, 1984; Pitt, 1968; Radloff & Rae, 1979). In such circumstances the mother may take a rejecting attitude toward the child or an excessively "needy" one. Either attitude can set up a maladaptive pattern of interaction between mother and child.

It appears, then, that increased knowledge coupled with adequate emotional resources may promote adaptive interaction patterns and enable teen mothers to be more effective parents. An examination of the means by which teens acquire childrearing knowledge and modify attitudes can yield a sense of the types of help that would be most appropriate for teen mothers.

TEACHING CHILDREN TO BE MOTHERS

Education appears to be somewhat more important than age in determining how, where, and when mothers seek childrearing help and information. In their 1985 study, Vukelick and Kliman found that the higher the mother's level of education the more varied and numerous were the sources she was likely to consult. Educated women tended to seek information during pregnancy and in advance of the appearance of any problems. They typically consulted written material—books, articles, or pamphlets. They also sought professional guidance fairly readily and were likely to discard erroneous beliefs if presented with contrary evidence. In contrast, less-educated mothers did not seek advice or information until a definite question or problem presented itself. They relied on fewer sources of information, usually confined to verbal advice from family, friends, or neighbors. They tended not to make use of printed materials, optional parenting classes, or professional advice.

Adolescents, simply by virtue of their age, have little education; furthermore, their life experience is limited. They are less accustomed to seeking out resources for themselves than older mothers are, and even when presented with information they may require help in applying it. Thus, teenage mothers tend to rely almost exclusively on their families, particularly their mothers and grandmothers, for information on child development and child care techniques. If an older sister or peer has children, she also may serve as an information source.

This evidence implies that if we seek to expand the knowledge base of young mothers it will not be sufficient simply to rely on school personnel or to make printed material available. Information will be better transmitted, and more likely absorbed and used, if it comes individually from a person who also maintains social contact with the teen. Ideally, contact with the teen's family may be desirable, to avoid or ameliorate a conflict between "our ways and their ways." In addition, the individual contact might be used to train the teen mother in more effective and sophisticated information seeking, need identification, and use of available community resources.

Similarly emotional and social variables may be modified. The above type of training may enhance competency and raise self-esteem. It may also aid in the development of new sources of social support. Particularly in segments of the culture in which adolescent parenthood is not the norm, the teenage mother may find herself lonely and isolated after her baby's birth. She is no longer free to indulge in many leisure activities; she no longer has much in common with her peers; she is cut off from the high school world yet does not fit in among other mothers who are 10 years her senior. The problem of peer support may be less acute in minority subgroups in which most of the other young girls also have children, but the temporal demands of motherhood still tend to preclude much social contact. The identification of new sources of social and practical support might prevent the loneliness and depression that would negatively affect the mother-child relationship.

In 1985 the author began a study to explore the roles of demographic, personality, support, and other variables in the outcome of teen parenthood. (This study is discussed more fully in chapters 4 and 5.) Of particular interest were the types of childrearing attitudes and practices displayed by young mothers and the relationship of these to the degree of social support and stress-coping resources available to the mother during and after her pregnancy. Two samples were used: One consisted to girls from a predominantly white, low-to-middle-income community in a suburb of a major city. The other sample contained girls from lower-income, largely black neighborhoods in an inner city. All the girls were pregnant or already parents at the beginning of the study; a few were pregnant for the second time. During the study, undergraduate university students were trained and assigned to work individually with the girls as peer advocates. The purpose was to offer social support and friendship to the girls, later to include informal, individual teaching in coping with adult responsibilities, such as budgeting and menu planning, in thinking futuristically about career and educational goals, and in seeking out and using resources in the community.

Data are as yet unavailable on the effects of the peer advocacy intervention. Preliminary data on the characteristics of the teen mothers in the study reveal surprising variations in knowledge and attitudes among the girls. Their levels of factual knowledge were quite low, despite training in child development and nutrition at their high schools. This suggests that the material presented in the classroom, no matter how effectively taught, will not generalize to actual behavior without reinforcement. This possibility is also worth noting as it affects sex education programs in schools— more than information may be required to encourage pregnancy prevention.

The girls attitudes toward their children display an apparent contradiction. During pretesting before the intervention began, the Block Child-rearing Practices Inventory, as revised by Rickel and Biasatti (1982), was administered to each girl. This questionnaire is designed to assess child-rearing attitudes that fall into two overall factors: nurturance and restrictiveness. Overall, the high school mothers scored high on both factors. Until more is known about how these attitudes are related to actual maternal behavior, it is difficult to interpret such results. They may represent very positive attitudes, on the order of providing firm but loving guidance. However, they might also represent the young mother's ego dependency on her baby. An overwhelming majority of the teens in the sample answered *yes* to such items as "I find may greatest satisfaction in my child" (a nurturance item), "I do not want my child to be seen as different from others" (restrictiveness), and "I would like my child to make a good impression on other people" (restrictiveness). Clearly much more evidence is needed before a sweeping conclusion can be drawn, but these tentative results suggest that the teen mothers in this sample pin most of their aspirations on their children and live through them to no small extent. This could lead to overly high expectations and demands on the children, which have been linked to later maternal frustration, disappointment, rejection, and in some cases child abuse (Isaacs, 1981). These girls clearly love and want their babies. However, the data suggest that they lack the resiliency to adapt to their children's individual needs. Rather, some of them may unrealistically expect their children to provide the love and sense of identity that they lack.

ADOLESCENT FATHERS

Most research on the parenting abilities of teens has focused exclusively on mothers, while adolescent fathers have received scant attention. There is a long-standing stereotype, both in popular thinking and, tacitly, in social science research, that teenage fathers are irresponsible, want nothing to do with their children, and generally desert their pregnant girlfriends. Undoubtedly this is true in many cases; however, it is equally possible that the stereotype becomes a self-fulfilling prophecy. Youthful fathers may not take on an active parenting role because they are discouraged from doing so or at least are not assisted in becoming good fathers. Few social services or mental health interventions aimed at teen parents include the fathers in any of their programs (Hamburg, 1986).

Familial pressure may cause the adolescent father to avoid the parent role. His own family might worry that their son will be entrapped by his girlfriend and child (Allen-Meares, 1984). They might wish to avoid financial responsibility for the child. Middle-class parents fear their son's loss of educational or career opportunities if he "ties himself down" with the child. The girl's family may blame her boyfriend for the pregnancy and reject him in anger; they could also separate the teens in order to punish the girl (Hamburg, 1986). They may not wish to share control of their daughter and grandchild (Furstenburg, 1980). The young mother herself might refuse to identify the father, for a variety of legal, financial, and personal reasons.

Cultural factors also work against effective teenage fatherhood. Our culture has a predilection toward viewing children as a women's concern, almost exclusively. Even the current media cry for responsibility among fathers addresses primarily issues of financial responsibility. Fathers are viewed as economic support and, unfortunately, little else, particularly as the feminization of poverty in single-parent homes has become common knowledge (Rivera-Casale, Klerman, & Manela, 1984). Some minority subcultures are basically matriarchal in structure, with a definite social barrier between males and females. In these subgroups childrearing and social support come only from the mother and her female kin, even in two-parent homes. Even married women do not regard their husbands as significant sources of emotional support (Hendricks, 1983).

There are, unquestionably, serious personal reasons for the avoidance of responsibility displayed by some high school fathers. Many simply do not wish to have their freedom curtailed. Among black teen fathers there appears to be greater acceptance of partial involvement with the mother and child, without the complete adoption of parental responsibility. Ironically, the young fathers most able to contribute to their children's upbringing are least likely to want to do it. Middle-class youth plan on going to college and developing their careers. They generally do not want to sacrifice this objective for parenthood. They are more likely than minority youth to regard abortion as an acceptable choice in pregnancy decision-making; thus, they believe that if the girl chooses not to avail herself of this option, she bears the responsibility for the child.

Despite all of the factors that work against the teenage father's participation in childrearing, there is some evidence that many of them do remain interested in their children and interact with them to varying degrees. Hendricks and Montgomery (1983) found that in a sample of black teen fathers in the Midwest, 98% expressed interest in their children's future and 60% reported being in love with the child's mother, both before and after the pregnancy. Hendricks (1983) found that teen fathers expressed a desire for guidance in their new parent role and felt left out because all the attention was centered on the mother. Boys tended to see themselves primarily in roles of social guidance and modeling, recreation, and, to a slightly lesser degree, material provisions (Eversoll, 1979). Girls expected them to take more of an active role in nurturance, physical care, and discipline than the boys thought they should. This disparity in role expectations clearly points out at least one area of possible intervention, since frustrated expectations would be a likely source of conflict and breakup for adolescent parents.

Possibly this self-definition of the father role among adolescent males may contribute to the parenting attitudes and behavioral statements that Johnson et al. (1982) noted in a sample of Iowa high school students. It was found that boys overall scored much lower than girls in knowledge of child behavior and development, with more inappropriately high expectations of children. The same study concluded that boys also had much more restrictive punitive attitudes in dealing with child behavior problems and were more likely to resort to physical force. Highlee (1981) found that, as a group, fathers see their children as less obedient than their mothers do. The possibility is raised that fathers are more exacting in their standards of obedience than are mothers. Feldman (1977) found that despite self-reported interest in children, males remained physically more distant from babies, looked at them less, and were less responsive to them than females were. The major implication of these studies is that better and earlier parent education and experience with children is called for if fathers are to take an active role as parents. There are suggestions (Johnson et al., 1982) that males are more likely than females to become child abusers and that appropriate education may be effective in preventing future abuse. Hendricks (1983) recommends a peer-counseling model designed to integrate the teen father into the social system as a parent over and above transmission of knowledge and skills.

Most teenage parent couples never marry each other, but teen mothers usually do become involved with other men later in life. No substantial research exists on the positive and negative roles these later male figures play in the children's lives. Presumably, personality variables in the mothers direct their choice of later partners, which then could mean either support or abuse for the child.

MARRIED TEENS

What of teen parents who do marry? The shotgun wedding was once the preferred solution to unwanted pregnancies, and many social factions now call for its return. The question remains as to whether any benefits other than legitimacy accrue to the child. There are several advantages; perhaps the greatest is that the child has a father present. One obvious problem is economics: Due to lack of education and restrictive labor laws, two teen-agers cannot earn enough to keep a family going. Under present law if a teen mother marries she loses eligibility for AFDC benefits. Parental support may also decrease, since marriage traditionally marks the entry into self-supporting adulthood. And although teens can legally marry in most states by age 15 or 16, they may not sign a lease or any other binding contract, receive credit, get a loan, or in many cases even authorize medical care until they reach 18. Emancipation of minority varies from state to state and often does not enable teen couples to live independently.

Adolescent marriages generally do not last more than 2 or 3 years (Carlson & Stinson, 1982). External stressors such as money take the heaviest toll. If the couple does live on their own, the stress is greater, and they risk social isolation—a major factor in domestic violence (Anderson & Lauderdale, 1982). Continuing to live with either the husband's or the wife's parents, however, may also produce conflicts and prevent full adult differentiation from the parents. Finally, there is evidence that most teens are not emotionally or cognitively prepared for marital commitment. They are still in the throes of the psychological upheaval of identity formation and emotional maturation; further, their ideas of adult life are unrealistic. Tamashiro (1979) identified five developmental stages in attitudes about marriage. There were no teens in his sample of 145 who had gone beyond the first two attitudes: magical and idealized. Early marriage, whether or not divorce follows, generally predicts lower educational and occupational attainment and lower income for the mothers even than single parenthood (Carlson & Stinson, 1982), probably because other supports are lost.

THE MATERNAL FAMILY AS ANTISUPPORT: DYSFUNCTIONAL FAMILY SYSTEMS

It is too often assumed that although the teen mother might need help in learning to handle the responsibilities of parenthood, generally all would be well for her child if her family assumed an active role in the care and support of the baby. In many cases that may be true. However, it often happens that the pregnancy occurs as one outcome of a disturbed or conflicted family situation. In such an instance it is reasonable to suppose that, far from curing the families' problems, new children may serve merely to continue them and to become both victims and transmitters of a disordered family dynamic, as were their mothers.

This possibility deserves particular consideration in light of the personality characteristics that have been linked to adolescent pregnancy, as discussed in the previous chapter. Low levels of self-esteem, aspiration, and self confidence; dependency, immaturity, and craving for attention; and impulsivity, acting out, and denial were among the traits common to large proportions of pregnant/parenting adolescents. Many of these traits are also common in children of dysfunctional homes, particularly those in which abuse, alcoholism, or immature parents are present. Likewise, several of these traits have been linked with the tendency to become abusive and/or alcoholic oneself. This suggests a generational chain of warped functioning: The family problems result in character factors that precipitate pregnancy; the girl and her child remain trapped in the maladaptive situation; the child is then at risk for later problems. The young mother may simply repeat the pattern set down by her parents; also, the grandparents' interaction with the baby is likely to be suboptimal or harmful.

An example of the cycle is that of the alcoholic family. When one or both parents are alcoholics, the children are likely to exhibit one of several adaptation styles (Black, 1979). Although these methods of coping may be necessary and constructive for the child, they nonetheless produce negative self-concept and behavior patterns that continue into adulthood. Black further states that among these coping styles is that of flight from the home and responsibility. It includes acting out and rebellious behavior, and a common outcome is teen pregnancy.

The first concern here is with the child who is partly raised by the alcoholic grandparent and thus suffers the same psychological fate as that of the teen mother. Thus, the cycle continues. Furthermore, alcoholism carries a familial component: Children of alcoholics are more likely than average to become alcoholics themselves and/or marry alcoholics (Black, 1979).

Children of alcoholics often carry emotional injuries that adversely affect their ability to form satisfying relationships. They tend to avoid discussing feelings and to have difficulty in honestly facing their own emotions. They have little self-esteem, confidence, or sense of worth. Often, they behave as emotional chameleons, adapting themselves to fit the situation. They have very low frustration tolerance and are controlled and responsible to excess or not at all, possibly displaying impulsive, reckless, irresponsible behavior. Finally, they are dominated by chronic fear, anxiety, depression, and long-simmering anger (*One day at a time in Al-Anon*, 1985).

It is obvious that these problems could interfere with the establishment of a satisfactory mother-child relationship. The tendency of these mothers to develop substance dependency themselves is also of obvious concern, not least because of the link between substance abuse and child abuse and neglect.

Most child abusers were themselves abused, molested, or neglected as children (Anderson & Lauderdale, 1982). Abused children generally reach adulthood with low self-esteem, low self-efficacy, unresolved anger and anxiety, and above all an unsatisfied longing for love and nurturance. Typically, abusive mothers had their children in the hopes that their babies would provide exclusive and limitless love, nurturance, affection, and approval. When, inevitably, a child proves unable to provide this and instead makes his or her own needs known, the mother often responds with anger, frustration, and disappointment—she strikes out at the child (Rieder, 1978).

In the previous chapter, various reasons why teens choose to get pregnant intentionally were discussed. One of the chief reasons given by young mothers is the craving for love. The baby is seen as a personal and exclusive source of affection and support. Intuitively, the inevitable result of disappointment and abuse is obvious. The empirical evidence makes it even more striking.

Thus, the double threat is clear: If the child's birth was the result of abusive or otherwise negative relations between the teen mother and her parents, then the child is threatened by the grandparents, who may treat the baby as they did his or her mother, and from the mother herself, who is likely to carry the pathological cycle on into her childrearing practices.

RISK FACTORS IN CHILD ABUSE

Teen mothers as a group are often regarded as high-potential child abusers, but the evidence for this is not conclusive (Kinard & Klerman, 1980). The greatest source of confounding appears to be the difficulty of controlling for socioeconomic status. Teen mothers who become known abusers tend to come from lower-socioeconomic-status groups. It appears likely that external stressors common to this group, such as economic stress, housing problems, unemployment, and crime, tax the coping resources of the mother and set the stage for abusive behavior in response to anxiety and frustration (McAdoo, 1985). However, it was noted that members of low-socioeconomic-status groups might be more likely to come to the attention of authorities as abusers, and the incidence of actual abuse may or may not be higher than in other socioeconomic-status groups. However, teen mothers, more than mature mothers, tend to experience high levels of economic-related stress by virtue of their lack of education and vocational skills (Isaacs, 1981).

External stress in general is linked to abuse (Isaacs, 1981; Ziglor & Rubin, 1985). Overwork and fatigue are common among single mothers, including teens, who work, parent, cope with household affairs, and often go to school. The effects of juggling tight schedules with no or few backup resources in case of emergency can be cumulative and quite deleterious to interaction within the family. Such schedules also leave little time for relaxed playtime or open communication.

Social isolation and loneliness have also been implicated as risk factors, and effective social support is believed to help prevent child abuse by mediating these factors (Barth & Schinke, 1984).

Often, child-related stress precipitates abuse. A colicky baby who screams all night for a week at a time may fall victim to the mother's maddened drive to stop the crying and get some rest. Children with physical/medical problems who require extra care similarly tax their mothers' patience. Parents may abuse developmentally delayed children who do not meet their expectations either out of frustration or in a misguided attempt to "teach" the child. Extremely active children, including but not limited to those diagnosed as hyperactive, tend to receive excessively punitive discipline that may become abusive. Finally, the more children there are and the more closely they are spaced, the higher the risk of abuse (Isaacs, 1981).

Many of these problems are among those to which children of teen mothers are especially prone. Their babies are at risk for low birth weight; lowered resistance to infection; and higher than average rates of slowed motor development, hyperactivity, academic retardation, peer socialization problems, and disciplinary problems. It appears then that those most at risk for having problem children are the least able to cope with the stresses involved (Barth & Schinke, 1984).

Teen mothers are faced with the task of learning to care for their children on three basic levels: physical care; guidance and discipline; and affection, nurturance, and support. Each of these areas is itself complex and requires many kinds of knowledge and problem-solving. There is good reason to question teen mothers' parenting abilities on each level and to suggest that different types of training are appropriate for each area.

Teens' performance in the area of physical care of their children appears quite variable. Some, particularly those who have the guidance and direction of older mothers or their own mothers, appear to do quite well. They have a good basic knowledge of child development, health, nutrition, and so forth and appear able to meet their children's physical needs fairly responsibly and consistently (Miller, 1984). However, significant numbers of adolescents are ignorant of babies' and children's physical needs and how to meet them (Johnson et al., 1982). Experience with younger siblings appears to be a poor predictor of child care skills. Moreover, a common feature of the adolescent generally is inconsistent performance, despite expressed desire to meet responsibilities. Thus, knowledge of child care practices and a desire to be an effective parent may be necessary but not sufficient for the establishment of consistently effective caregiving in adolescent mothers. The conflicting evidence regarding teens' ability to care for children probably represents differences among mothers attributable to factors other than knowledge and childrearing attitudes alone. Further research is needed to determine what factors promote sound caregiving in young mothers.

Most studies of teen parents' discipline practices center on the mothers' response to child misbehavior. Johnson et al. (1982) found that older girls tend to respond with reinforcement of good behavior, time out, or similar corrective rather than punitive techniques more frequently than younger girls. It is known that younger children view misbehavior more harshly and respond more punitively than do older youngsters and adults. Further, some adolescents display a tendency to discipline more on the basis of their emotional reaction to the child's behavior at a given moment, rather than any objective criterion of the acceptability of the behavior (Kinard & Klerman, 1980). The response of LaDawn, in the case study at the beginning of this chapter, exemplifies this type of response. LaDawn disciplines only if her child angers her; she acts according to her mood more than to the child's actions. Inconsistent discipline of this type may bring with it a variety of problems, not the least of which is absence of any real behavioral control of the child, who quickly learns to second-guess his mother's mood. Juvenile behavior problems in school and community settings may result.

The practice of child discipline does not, however, begin and end with response to misbehavior; rather, it involves establishing rules and setting general standards of conduct. Little or no research has been done regarding the ability of teen mothers to set standards for their children and transmit them effectively. Roosa (1984) found that young parents tend to be somewhat inconsistent in their parenting attitudes and put them into practice inconsistently. This suggests that it is questionable whether adolescents are equipped to function adequately as rule-setters for their children.

Much of the research on the child care practices of teen mothers has focused on the aspect of nurturance as seen through mother-infant interactions. Research indicates that teen mothers may show affection to their infants as much as, or more than, older mothers; however, they tend to stimulate them less. Landy, Schubert, Cleland, Clark, and Montgomery (1983) found that young teen mothers looked at their babies' faces less often, smiled less, and directed less vocalization to their infants in comparison to older mothers. Teen mothers hug and kiss their babies more but play with them less and spend more time in physical care activities. They tend to leave their babies in the crib for longer periods of time. Landy et al.'s description suggests a highly nurturant attitude on the part of the young mothers, but also that the mothers regard their children almost as dolls—something to hug rather than to teach and interact with. This may help explain King and Fullard's (1982) observation that teen mothers frequently feel caring toward their children, satisfied with their children's and their own behavior, and competent in their maternal role, yet interact with their children in minimal or unsatisfactory ways. King and Fullard further found evidence suggestive of cultural differences in normal childrearing habits: They found higher restrictiveness and less verbal interaction in minority samples than in white samples; this probably reflects both cultural and socioeconomic differences. Large individual differences were also found, suggesting that teens acquire the ability to put attitudes into practice to a greater or lesser extent depending on a host of other variables.

It is notable that most mother-child interaction studies have focused on teen mothers' responsiveness to infants. Longitudinal studies of mothers' interaction with their older children are lacking. Kinard and Reinherz (1984) found that, despite some physical/maturational difficulties experienced by children of teen mothers, they do not show significantly different verbal development or behavioral problems by age 6 in comparison with other children. The implication of this for individual differences in childrearing patterns and the differences between factors affecting the mother-child relationship and those affecting the child's development are still to be assessed. The prevailing assumption that certain features of mother-child interaction have long-term effects on child development may be mediated by cultural and other factors.

In the foregoing discussion of teen parents' childrearing practices, it becomes apparent that education and socioeconomic status are more powerful determinants of maternal behavior than age alone (Landy, Cleland, & Schubert, 1984). This suggests that education generally, apart from specific parent training, is likely to have an ameliorative effect on the problems of early parenthood.

EDUCATION AND JOB TRAINING

Education promotes positive parenting in its most direct and obvious way when it results in improved knowledge of child care and development and improved attitudes toward parenting. As Johnson et al. (1982), Roosa (1984), and others attest, improved mother-child interactions can be promoted directly through parent-training programs aimed at high school mothers.

More indirect benefits are observed from the attainment of higher overall levels of education. Better-educated mothers provide more stimulation, more appropriate toys, a more orderly home environment, more consistent rules, more encouragement in independent efforts, and more stability than less-educated mothers (Blum, 1984; King & Fullard, 1982). They rely on more sources of support and are more likely to seek outside help—medical, social, and other—for themselves and their children than less-educated women (Vukelick & Kliman, 1985). Parent behavior is also a function of self-esteem and self-efficacy, which are influenced positively by increased levels of education (Blum, 1984).

Perhaps the major benefit of education is that it helps to raise the mothers' socioeconomic status. In cases in which early childbearing sinks the young mother into poverty or prevents her from leaving it, the child suffers not only from material deprivation but also the social and educational problems of growing up in the underclass (Blum, 1984; Delatte, Orgeron, & Preis, 1985). The financial, housing, transportation, crime, and other problems of poor mothers create stresses that may result in child maltreatment (Isaacs, 1981). When family support is available to the young mother and child, poverty may be avoided, but the girl will be unable to ever live independently without education (Barth & Schinke, 1984).

Education is necessary but not always sufficient for obtaining full and decent employment. Failure to complete high school has been shown to be predictive of long-term welfare dependency and poverty (Blum, 1984). This is likely to be ever more the case as the United States shifts from a unionized manufacturing economy toward one split between highly paid white-collar workers and very poorly paid service workers (Ruffin, 1986). Recently, there has been a tremendous increase in the number of entry-level and unskilled jobs available (Sheets, 1986). However, these jobs are insecure, to say the least; they are in the most volatile segments of the American market. They are dead-end jobs without promotion opportunities or benefits, mostly in food service industries (Nilsen, 1985). They pay minimum wage, which is rarely sufficient to support a mother and child, and many of these jobs may soon be paid a subminimum youth wage, geared to teens who want to earn pocket money rather than to young parents (Carpenter, 1985; Donovan, Hawkins, Hatch, Clay, Dixon, Tucker, Donison, Welch, & O'Hara, 1985; Rankin, 1985; Ruffin, 1984). Despite the much-discussed need for new workers, many of these jobs still elude young people, due to lack of even rudimentary skills, lack of transportation, and a host of other problems (McCarthy, 1986; Butler, 1986). Even if *immediate* employment is available, in the long run teens and their children are better off if the mother forgoes income from full-time work long enough to complete her schooling (Blum, 1984; Feather & O'Brien, 1986). A current problem is that a high school diploma or the equivalency is no longer enough as a credential for a first job. Some specialized technical training, college, or business apprenticeship is necessary, particularly in areas open to women. Many cooperative and peer-mentor programs have proven successful in keeping young mothers in high school (Atkinson, 1986; Blum, 1984; Delatte et al., 1985; Harrison, 1987; Turkel & Abramson, 1986; Campbell, 1987). Perhaps even more crucial to the eventual socioeconomic status of young single parents is the special training now being offered by many businesses; these programs have greatly reduced youth unemployment (Dreyfuss, 1985; Hale, 1986; Olson, Smith, & Farkas, 1986; Sharples, 1986).

Employment affects much more than the children's material well-being. Employed single mothers (those not in school) experience less financial stress, less worry, and less depression than unemployed mothers (Polit, 1987). They have more sense of control over their lives, higher frustration tolerance, and higher self-esteem (Tiggaman & Winefield, 1984). These factors make them less likely to become pregnant again (Barth & Schinke, 1984) and less likely to abuse substances (Black, 1979) or to abuse or neglect their children (Isaacs, 1981; Anderson & Lauderdale, 1982). They tend to engage in more nurturant, more attentive/supervisory, stimulating, and less restrictive parent behaviors, which increases their children's self-esteem (Weigle, 1976). These factors have been related to more empathy and better moral reasoning in children, better socialization, internal control, and motivation to achieve (Wilkinson & O'Connor, 1977). Employment that raises the socioeconomic status of the mother also increases the likelihood of such desirable maternal attitudes and practices as low restrictiveness, high nurturance and stimulation, and greater verbal communication (King & Fullard, 1982). Employed mothers are generally able to provide more stability in the home environment than mothers who depend on public assistance (Barber, Cernetig, Geddes, Smith, Steacy, Lord, Van Dusen, Jones, & Lowthor, 1986; Daniels, 1986).

All of the above considerations regarding the importance of education, training, and job placement in the ability to parent apply as much to teen fathers as to mothers. Teen fathers encounter many of the same employment problems that girls do: With or without a high school diploma, unemployment among youth is high (Williams, 1984). Available jobs pay only minimum wage, unless the boy obtains marketable skills (Lewis, 1985). And teen fathers are more likely than nonfathers to be high school dropouts and to have low aspirations; they also share with the mothers such characteristics as external locus of control, which places them at risk for underachievement (Hendricks & Montgomery, 1983). Thus, efforts to involve adolescent fathers in the support and care of their children must involve efforts to encourage them to complete at least a high school education and to obtain some further training in job skills. This is a particularly important issue in the inner cities, where youth unemployment soars well over 60% (Anderson, 1987; Holden, 1985).

Lack of day care is a persistent problem encountered by teen mothers attempting to complete school or hold a job. Often the girl's mother takes on child care duties; the costs and benefits of this arrangement have been described earlier. However, depending on other friends and relatives can carry with it both logistical and emotional/interpersonal stress. Further, informal sources of child care are not always available on a consistent basis. Day care centers are in short supply and often have long waiting lists. Transportation is frequently a major problem for teens. Finally, the cost of day care is often prohibitive; many single mothers are on welfare because they cannot earn enough to obtain child care (Harrison, 1985). The day care that is available to low-income mothers is often of poor quality. Thus, children of teen mothers may be left unsupervised and often suffer neglect (Miller, 1984). Mothers may, on the other hand, remain at home out of concern for their children's safety.

For the young teen mother, reliable, low-cost, quality day care may be the magic ingredient that permits her to complete school. Alternative education programs in some school systems offer free onsite day care for high school mothers. These programs keep many young mothers in school and may also provide them with a source of information about good child-rearing practices, child health and development, and referrals to other service providers (Harrison, 1987; Schmidt, 1985). Not all schools have such services, however, and in some systems they are available only at alternative schools and for limited periods of time. When teen mothers are mainstreamed back to their home schools, they may drop out for lack of day care and other services. Some may get pregnant again in order to remain in the alternative program (Rickel, Montgomery, Thomas, Butler, Meade, & Rowland, 1988). School-based day care appears to be a key tool in promoting the welfare of teen mothers and their children. It would seem to also offer an ideal "laboratory" for high school parent training classes.

Adoption once was almost the only option, other than marriage, available to teens who became pregnant. Now fewer than 10% of pregnant teens even seriously consider adoption. Various reasons have been offered as an explanation. The availability of abortion has cut the percentage of teen pregnancies carried to term by a wide margin. Subcultural taboos against giving up one's child exert pressure on teens. Popular lore has it that this taboo is particularly strong in the black and Hispanic communities, although the evidence for this idea is mixed (Mech, 1986). The decision about pregnancy resolution may be influenced by a girl's parents and by her peers (Rickel, et al., 1988). However, the teen who chooses to have a baby clearly has no intention of giving the child up. Mech (1986) asserts that this trend is also the result of counselors who simply assume that adoption will not be considered and do not even explore the subject with the pregnant teen. His research suggests, rather convincingly, that increased availability of information concerning adoption and adoptive homes might result in increased placement of babies with adoptive parents in cases where the young mother feels unable to provide adequately for the child. Concern for the baby's future welfare was, in Mech's study, the only consideration that prompted a strong interest in adoption on the part of the pregnant teens.

Such considerations are important given what is known about the difficulties of teen parenthood. The characteristics of the teens who choose to abort have been compared with those who carry their pregnancies to term (Olson, 1980). Overall, those who abort tend to be of high socioeconomic status; their aspirations and career goals are high; they are more likely to complete school; and they have higher self-esteem, more internal locus of control, fewer emotional disturbances, and more stable families than girls who carry their pregnancies to term. Additionally, those girls who become pregnant intentionally generally do so for less-than-adaptive reasons: as social acting out, to hurt parents, to conform to peers, to get attention and love, to get emotional support from the child, or to gain a sense of achievement. It thus becomes apparent that, of all girls who get pregnant, those who actually have the baby are those least able to parent effectively.

Many of the children of these girls come to the attention of community child protective services, either through abuse or neglect. Some of the main determinants of out-of-home placement in foster care for these children are parental stress factors, parental problem behaviors such as substance abuse, and stability of relationships in the family, to name a few. On many of these dimensions, children of teen mothers may be at risk for placement in foster care (Ratterman, 1986). Foster care seldom ends in adoptive homes for older children. Rather, it often is the beginning of a long series of moves to numerous environments of questionable quality and little stability (Brenner, 1985; Sudia, 1986). Reducing stress factors for teen mothers, enhancing social supports and coping skills, and training mothers in parenting techniques obviously may help prevent many children from becoming foster care cases. However, in cases where the young mother-to-be is ambivalent or negative about the prospect of parenthood, efforts should be made to increase the availability of adoption placement.

For any mother to contemplate permanent separation from her baby is very difficult. Open adoption arrangements are an attempt to ease this process for the new mother by allowing visitation with the child and the adoptive family, even, in a few cases, going so far as to allow split custody of the child. Such arrangements are now being tried in several states (Waddill, 1984). Long-term results will not be available for several years; however, the plan has intuitive merits. It frees more children for adoption, gives the children the advantage of a mature home, and allows the girl to pursue her education and life plans; yet it does not require that the mother and baby be forever separated and unknown to each other.

CHILDREN HAVING CHILDREN—HOW WE CAN HELP THEM GROW UP

Most older societies have had some rite of passage that clearly marked the transition to adulthood. Western culture lacks such a boundary point, and in modern times the ever-increasing length of adolescence brings with it conflict and confusion about when and how to confer adulthood on the individual. The phenomenon of teen parenthood forces us as a society to make some hard decisions about how we define adulthood and what, if anything, we will do to prepare youth for it. In the United States one is legally an adult at age 18; yet many (or most) 18-year-olds are still in high school, generally considered a state in which we expect people to behave as kids. After high school, then, one might expect people to formally take on adult identity. Yet little in their experience has trained them for this. Familial role models are often absent. Since women's roles are changing rapidly, it is difficult for girls to find an effective model. The media offers utterly unrealistic portraits of adult life. High school, as mentioned before, is frequently viewed only as an entryway to college and teaches little in the way of adult living skills, decision-making, and the like. Finally, economics have forced a lengthening of "social" adolescence, sometimes into the mid 20s, while college degrees are obtained and budding careers started. Because the relative cost of living has risen dramatically in the last 10 years, many young adults remain in the parental home for financial reasons. In a society that has traditionally defined leaving home as a necessary step to adulthood, this may cause some identity confusion on all sides. Another traditional rite of passage, marriage, may be delayed or omitted altogether. Education is a protracted affair; this trend may have some negative effects in the form of increased emotional dependency and lessened self-worth and sense of identity in dependent students over age 20, compared to age-peers who are self-supporting nonstudents. Thus, adulthood in America may be overly delayed (Hamburg, 1986).

One function is and has always been considered sacrosanct in itself and a prerogative of adulthood: childbearing and childrearing. Parental rights supersede other considerations, except in cases of marked danger to the child. Thus, teen pregnancy confers only *partial* adulthood on the girl. She cannot vote, drink a beer, or hold a job; she may not even be permitted to drive a car, but she is entrusted with raising a child. She would not normally be permitted to bind herself in a contract, but she may make serious decisions for her child. Marriage laws reflect this ambiguity: In some states a girl as young as 13 may marry, although she is supposedly not an adult until years later.

These contradictions and ambiguities have long been with us and are pointed out here for the sake of illustration. No one would reasonably suggest that higher education is undesirable or that legal majority should begin at puberty! But it does raise the issue of how we might best use the middle and high school years to ease youth into adulthood, rather than barring them from it. It is suggested that training for *all* students, from middle school up, in life skills, career management, childrearing, and vocational possibilities could have important effects. It may enable teen parents to function more effectively by giving them the skills and confidence they need before they actually become parents, and it could facilitate changes in the social network by preventing the teen parent from becoming barred from teen society. It may also complement sex education programs by giving students more confidence, self-esteem, and self-efficacy; more realistic ideas of adult and parenting roles; and experience in goal-setting, decision-making, and responsible action. Thus, preparing kids to be adults might actually result in fewer teen pregnancies.

Chapter 3

High-Risk Infants and Teen Mothers

Despite efforts to abate the rising incidence of adolescent motherhood, teens continue to give birth at alarming rates. This picture is complicated by the fact that families most vulnerable to poverty are those headed by women, and, because of the greater stress to which these mothers are subjected, children in female-headed households show more impairment (Ford Foundation Report, 1983). Where prevention of pregnancy has failed, one must address the pressing needs of infants born to this group of young, inexperienced mothers.

Infants at risk include a large group of children who may be disadvantaged due to problematic reproductive outcomes or as a result of less than optimal caretaking practices (Field, 1982). Pasamanick and Knobloch (1961) described the *reproductive causality continuum* as a range of pre- and perinatal risk factors, such as congenital heart defects, intellectual deficits, prematurity, and low birth weight. The caretaking continuum, on the other hand, includes those developmental delays or difficulties that the child experiences as a direct result of his or her caretaking environment. Unfortunately, offspring of adolescent parents are often at risk due to both types of causalities.

THE CONTINUUM OF REPRODUCTIVE CAUSALITY

Three major areas of influence make up the reproductive causality continuum: heredity or genetic predispositions, pre- and perinatal factors surrounding the growth of the fetus and delivery of the infant, and the socioeconomic or environmental factors in which the child is raised.

Hereditary Factors

Size, appearance, intelligence, and muscular coordination are all in some measure genetically determined for humans. Further, it is now understood that emotional adjustment is in part determined at conception. Single gene defects such as PKU and sickle cell anemia have obvious implications for emotional adjustment. Although the link is less well understood and more complex, emotional thought disorders and disturbances such as schizophrenia and manic-depressive conditions are also genetically influenced (Roberts & Peterson, 1984).

Pre- and Perinatal Influences

Pre- and perinatal factors known to increase an infant's developmental risk include maternal illness, malnutrition, and use of alcohol and drugs. Prematurity, the outcome of many teen pregnancy complications, represents the most common birth abnormality. The adverse long-term impact of prematurity may be due to the shortened gestation alone or to associated factors, for example, concomitant perinatal trauma, low birth weight, a lengthy period of hospital incubation, or low socioeconomic conditions to which the child is exposed while growing up. Parmelee and Haber (1973) argue that premature infants who are reared in a warm, stimulating environment may fare just as well as full-term infants brought up under the same conditions. Goldberg (1979) has suggested that some of the developmental difficulties of premature infants may be related to interference in the establishment of parent-infant bonding. For example, mother-infant responsiveness may be inhibited by the preterm infant's lack of integrated physiologic and motoric functioning (Als, Tronick, & Lester, 1977). To combat this, Siqueland (1973) found that early intervention with premature infants enhanced the infants' ability to evoke more responsive interaction from their mothers.

Premature delivery has a tremendous emotional impact on the infant's parents, sometimes impairing their ability to adequately care for the newborn. Further, it is suggested that the future functioning of preterm infants may be determined to a large extent by factors unrelated to the specific impairment of the infant. This is of particular concern in teenage pregnancy where adolescent parents often lack the emotional resources to deal effectively with the many difficulties surrounding prematurity. Thus, any physical impairment measurable at birth is actually an inefficient predictor of the future overall functioning of these infants. Sigman and Parmelee (1979) found that it was actually the attitudes and child care practices of premature infants' caregivers that were the best predictors of the child's later development and adjustment.

Socioeconomic Conditions

Risk factors on the reproductive causality continuum are influenced by ethnic background and low social status. For instance, infant mortality rates have been found to be highest among women who are both poor and black. Complication rates, while only 5% for white upper-class groups, increase dramatically among all nonwhites (U.S. Bureau of the Census, 1982). It appears that in addition to less than optimal biological outcomes at birth, disadvantaged children experience less favorable developmental outcomes as well (Birch & Gussow, 1970).

Werner, Bierman, and French (1971) examined the effects of birth complications and socioeconomic status on child development in their classic longitudinal study. Physical development and psychological development were impaired in 20-month-old infants who had experienced perinatal complications only when they were subjected to poor environmental conditions after birth. Further, Werner et al. found that when good prenatal care was available to poor women the initial differences in the distribution of birth complications disappeared.

On reassessment of the children at 10 years of age (Werner & Smith, 1977), correlations between parent and child IQs were found to have increased over the first 8 years of life. This suggests that risk factors arising from perinatal complications wane during childhood under family and social influences. Werner and Smith reported that 10 times more children suffered intellectual, physical, or behavioral problems as a result of a disadvantaged early environment than from the impact of perinatal problems.

It is thus apparent that socioeconomic factors play a role in both reproductive and caretaking causalities. While socioeconomic status affects genetic and pre- and perinatal outcomes, the residual effects of complications also depend to a large extent on the socioeconomic conditions of the caretaking environment (Rickel & Allen, 1987).

THE CARETAKING CAUSALITY CONTINUUM

Included in the caretaking causality continuum are postnatal risk factors associated with early parenting practices. Caretaking behaviors that do not meet the minimum requirements for a child's healthy development place the child at risk for a number of caretaking causalities. Disturbed parent-child relationships may take many forms; however, child abuse and neglect have been the focus of much attention in recent years, particularly in regard to adolescent parenting (Sameroff & Chandler, 1975).

Maltreating Parents

Researchers have been interested in the characteristics or personality traits of abusive parents in an effort to identify parents who would have a propensity toward maltreatment of their children. Higher levels of anxiety and defensiveness were found in one group of abusive parents, who exhibited lower nurturance than control parents (Egeland, Breitenbucher, & Rosenberg, 1980). In their 1984 study, Lahey, Conger, Atkeson, and Treiber found battering parents to be of lower intelligence and more impulsive, self-centered, depressed, aggressive, and emotionally and somatically distressed than nonabusing parents.

A popular notion today is that parents who are abusive were themselves mistreated as children, learning maladaptive parenting habits through modeling. Rosenberg and Reppuci (1983) found parents such as these to be more critical of their childrearing abilities and practices than parents demonstrating more nurturant attitudes.

Another precursor of abuse and neglect is thought to be excessive socioenvironmental stress experienced by parents (Garbarino, 1976). In an attempt to isolate specific environmental stresses that might lead to abuse, Justice and Duncan (1976) examined stress-inducing events relative to a family's history. Far greater levels of stress (defined as a life change requiring adaptive action) were found to exist among abusing parents than among nonabusive control groups. Thus, the researchers concluded that specific life crises, rather than general stress related to socioeconomic conditions, were responsible for harsh, maladaptive forms of parenting.

In a similar study, Egeland and Brunquell (1979) identified a group of mothers who were found to mistreat their children between birth and 2 years of age. When compared to a matched group of mothers administering adequate care to their children, abusive/neglecting mothers were found to have experienced no greater number of stressful life events. However, it was noted that the severity of stressful events (degree of disruption and readjustment required) was much higher for maltreating mothers.

As a follow-up to these findings, Egeland et al. (1980) created a modified version of the Life Events Inventory developed by Cochrane and Robertson (1973). Using the new instrument they were able to differentiate between a group of abusive, maltreating mothers and nonabusive mothers on the basis of the total number of stressful life events experienced. Thus, it appears that life tension and stress do contribute to the presence of child neglect or violent behavior in the home.

Abused and Neglected Children

Offspring of adolescent mothers, as discussed earlier, are at risk for prematurity, perinatal complications, low birth weight, and congenital defects. Drotar, Malone, Negray, and Dennstedt (1981) found these characteristics to be overrepresented among abused/neglected children. Crittenden (1983) suggests that for parents who may be predisposed to mistreating their children the presence of unusual congenital conditions may increase the likelihood that they will succumb to abusive or neglectful parenting practices.

There is some evidence that children who are abused and mistreated have in some way contributed to their misfortune. For example, Morse, Sahler, and Friedman (1970) studied a group of 55 children who had been neglected or abused in some manner. Over 40% of the children were mentally impaired and/or hyperactive prior to the incidence of abuse. Similarly, Baldwin and Oliver (1975) found that children who exhibited developmental delays were prone to abusive treatment by parents. In 1970, Gil reported that almost one third of the mistreated children in his nationwide study had disturbed social relationships during the year prior to their physical or emotional abuse. Twenty-five percent had abnormal intellectual or physical functioning, and parents indicated that many of the children had consistently displayed atypical behavior.

Abused and neglected children are often described by parents as difficult, noncompliant, whiny, avoidant, unappealing, and clingy. In addition, they often have finicky eating habits (Robert & Maddux, 1982). Thus, parents of these children often report that their abusive behavior was provoked by their children. Crittenden (1983), on the other hand, suggests that the difficult and passive interaction patterns of neglected and abused infants may be a result of maltreatment rather than a cause.

To test this hypothesis, Crittenden videotaped infants while they interacted with their mothers and then with a second familiar adult. The infant was noted to produce the same pattern of behavior when both the mother and second adult had the same pattern of interaction. However, the infant's behaviors were observed to change when the second adult varied interaction patterns.

Ainsworth, Blehar, Waters, and Wall (1978) have posited that when parents are emotionally unavailable or physically reject their infants a pattern of anxious-avoidant attachment results. In the Crittenden study described above, a consistent pattern of serious maltreatment and anxious attachment was found. Further, Crittenden observed that adequate caregiving led to secure attachment, while marginal treatment produced mixed results.

Recently completed longitudinal research in New York City (Rickel

& Langner, 1985) suggests a clear association between marital disruption and child abuse as well as deficits in children's intellectual development and delinquency. Since so many adolescents are opting to rear their infants alone, one of the most pressing issues for the future is how to enhance the teen mother's parenting skills and thus promote a positive impact on the child's development.

PREVENTIVE INTERVENTIONS WITH HIGH-RISK INFANTS

Preconception Counseling

An early form of intervention prior to a planned conception is genetic counseling. Although its application to adolescent pregnancy is limited, its utility as a preventive strategy is great when known risk factors are present in the parents' medical histories. In genetic counseling the probability of a couple's future offspring inheriting specific disorders is determined and presented to the parents. In addition, the implications of various disorders are discussed in terms of the social, psychological, and financial costs to family members. While not directly involved in the decision-making process, the counselor is available to assist the couple in making an informed decision regarding conception. In a study assessing the effectiveness of genetic counseling, over one third of the couples who had been advised that their offspring would be at high risk for genetic disorders continued to pursue conception. In these cases it is assumed that the parents were able to take an informed risk, forearmed with awareness of the difficulties they might face.

Aiding Parents of Premature Infants

Prematurity is a crisis with which many teenage mothers must cope. In 1980, Widmayer and Field designed an intervention program to assist young black mothers of lower socioeconomic status and their preterm infants. In a previous study, Field (1980) noted that adolescent mothers tended to treat their infants like dolls who could not see or hear. The goal of the Widmayer and Field study, therefore, was to increase the mothers' verbal responsiveness to their infants by demonstrating the various skills of the newborn.

Two-person intervention teams made biweekly home visits with the goal of educating mothers about child development and childrearing techniques. In addition, they attempted to enhance the infants' cognitive and sensorimotor development while facilitating mother-infant interactions. Follow-up measures revealed that intervention participants performed better than controls on infant weight, length, Denver Developmental Scores, and face-to-face interactions. The mothers, in turn, showed realistic developmental expectations, displayed more extensive interactions with their infants, reported less punitive childrearing attitudes, and rated their infants' temperament as less difficult than did control mothers.

A hospital-based intervention that used peer-oriented self-help groups was designed by Minde, Shosenberg, and Marton (1982) to aid mothers of premature infants. Parents met once a week in small groups for approximately 7 to 12 weeks after the birth of their child. The groups were led by a neonatal nurse, and each group included a mother who had given birth to a premature infant within the last year.

The group format provided an opportunity for parents to discuss fears, guilt, and depression associated with their infant's prematurity. Additionally, parents were shown films and slides demonstrating the developmental and medical needs of premature infants. Group members were assisted with such practical matters as obtaining unemployment compensation and improved housing and finding babysitters. Social services were discussed, and participants were familiarized with local community services for family support.

Interestingly, families who participated in the discussion groups visited their infants in the hospital more often than the control parents (Minde, Shosenberg, Marton, Thompson, Ripley, & Burns, 1980). They rated themselves as more confident in their ability to care for their infants and touched and talked with their babies more often during visits. Group differences were maintained upon 3-month follow-up when discussion group mothers reported being more concerned about general developmental issues and were more actively involved with their infants during feedings.

Minde, Shosenberg, and Thompson (1983) performed a 1-year follow-up study that, again, revealed differences between intervention and control mothers. Experimental mothers were found to talk and play with their children more and were able to share their feelings with them more easily. They also gave their children greater freedom. From a self-image vantage point, mothers who had participated in discussion groups showed a more positive attitude toward their work, had a higher degree of personal autonomy, and reported their relationships with other people had improved. The children of these mothers displayed greater social development than did controls, exhibiting such independent behaviors as general playing, self-feeding, and food sharing. The authors suggest that the enriched interactions with their infants may in part be due to mothers' improved self-concepts.

Social-Psychological Interventions

The Pittsburgh First-Born Project (Broussard, 1982) focused specifically on the prevention of disorders of a social-psychological nature. High-risk infants were identified based on mothers' responses to the Neonatal Perception Inventories. This instrument asks new mothers to compare their newborn with the "average" infant. Children considered to be at risk are those whose mothers do not rate them as better than average during the first month of life. Broussard found the absence of positive maternal perceptions of the neonate to be associated with high rates of psychosocial disorders as children mature.

All children involved in the study were physically healthy and the first-born child in the family. The intervention consisted of mother-infant group meetings and in-home visits beginning when the infants were 2 to 3 months old and continuing for 3½ years. Mother-infant interactions were studied carefully, and each dyad received interventions specific to its needs. Reassessments of the children were undertaken at 1 and 2½ years of age. Results indicated that intervention children, as compared with control subjects, exhibited superior functioning in all of the following areas: confidence, coping, separation-individuation, aggression, affective balance, implementation of contacts with the nonhuman environment, investment in the use of language for communication, and play.

Interventions for Abusive and Maltreating Mothers

Crittenden and Snell (1983) reported on an intervention program designed for abusive and neglecting mothers of low socioeconomic status. Patterns of mother-infant interaction were assessed by means of videotaped play sessions. Maternal interaction was classified as being abusing, neglecting, inept, or sensitive. Similarly, infants' interaction was rated as passive, difficult, or cooperative. A developmental delay measure was also obtained.

The intervention itself consisted of weekly meetings at which each mother was again videotaped while interacting with her child. Together the group watched the tapes and discussed ways in which interactions could be improved. When children were reassessed after 4 months, it became clear that maternal patterns of mother-child interaction were related to maltreatment. Specifically, when the mother's interaction with her child was abusive, the infant's behavior was classified as difficult; when the mother was neglecting, the infant was passive; and when the maternal pattern of interaction was inept or sensitive, the infant was rated as cooperative. The highest developmental quotients (DQs) were found among infants of adequate or marginally maltreating mothers. Neglected infants had the lowest DQs.

One hypothesis of the study was that the infants would become more cooperative and show developmental gains as their mothers increased in their sensitivity to the child's needs. Infants did, in fact, become more cooperative in the majority of cases where the mother had shown an increase in sensitivity. Similarly, infant increases in DQs were found to be related to maternal sensitivity increases. Thus, Crittenden and Snell concluded that maltreatment is not a result of difficult infant behavior or temperament. Rather, aberrant mother-child interactions are initiated by the mother and then maintained by the infant's behavior. The study provides evidence that neglected and abused infants have the capacity for normal behavior when their mother's behavior moves in a positive direction.

Infants at Risk for Academic Failure

Based on a general systems model, the Carolina Abecedarian Project (Ramey & Campbell, 1981) focused on conditions affecting the growth of infants and children at risk for academic failure. Children in the experimental group received educational programming through day care as early as 6 weeks of age. The goals of the program were to facilitate concept attainment, language development, and adaptive social behavior in a supportive and predictable environment. Follow-up assessments at 6, 12, and 18 months revealed that experimental children exhibited greater social confidence, less fearfulness, an increased ability to execute abstract and complex tasks, and enhanced psycholinguistic skills. Further, they did not demonstrate the intellectual decline observed in control children.

In sum, a wide variety of risk factors associated with infancy have been successfully ameliorated through target intervention programs. Although some infant risk factors are unavoidable, many of the variables associated with risk in infancy are created directly or indirectly by parental childrearing practices and attitudes. Thus, the success of many interventions possibly rests on the fact that they not only provide stimulation to the child but also promote parental change through (a) parent education of child development; (b) increasing parents' self-image and their sense of childrearing competence; (c) providing supportive peer discussion groups; (d) enhancing parent-infant interactions in an effort to augment the child's social, emotional, and cognitive development; and (e) alerting parents to the availability of social services and encouraging their use of such resources (Rickel & Allen, 1987).

Chapter 4

Research Findings from Working with Pregnant Teens in the Public School System

BACKGROUND

Over the past several years the author has been involved in developing and evaluating a preventive/early intervention program for young children (The Preschool Mental Health Program). The program was initially funded by local foundations and the Detroit Public Schools, and in its first phase it provided services to preschool-age children. An intensive screening program using standardized pediatric, neurological, and achievement tests and social-emotional scales was implemented in the Detroit Public Schools, Region 7, for disadvantaged preschool children. Children were identified as high risk if they were experiencing learning or behavioral problems, and prescriptive remedial activities were developed for each child. Teachers and paraprofessionals were trained by the project staff to provide the remediation (Rickel, 1982). A training manual was also developed to aid in the intervention efforts (Rickel, 1979). Pre- and posttest measures have consistently indicated significantly improved performance for experimental children compared with randomly assigned placebo controls (Rickel &

Smith, 1979; Rickel, Smith, & Sharp, 1979). A 2-year follow-up evaluation further revealed that children who received the remediation sustained their gains as they moved into the primary grades in school (Rickel & Lampi, 1981).

THE DETROIT PARENT TRAINING PROJECT

A major objective of the Preschool Mental Health Project was to extend the influence of the project into the home by means of a parent training program. This extension was as much a research endeavor as it was a program of service delivery. As such, the program was an effort to gain a greater understanding of how to conduct an effective training program in parenting techniques.

The initial training program consisted of five consecutive weekly sessions and a follow-up session of approximately 2½ hours, each of which utilized a behavioral intervention approach. These sessions were held at the local school during regular school hours. At each session the group leaders introduced the topics, which included the importance of listening to children, how to handle the expression of a child's anger, children's fights, and appropriate discipline techniques. Parents were generally instructed in what is typical and atypical behavior for a preschool child. Techniques for dealing with inappropriate child behaviors were explained. Handout sheets outlining the most important points discussed in each session were also distributed, and parents were given a notebook for keeping the handouts and additional notes they might have taken in the sessions or at home.

The majority of time in each session was used for having parents practice the concepts that were presented through behavioral techniques. These included role playing, behavioral rehearsal, modeling, cognitive reshaping, and videotape feedback. Since for most parents these were new experiences, every effort was made to help the parents feel comfortable in discussing their thoughts and feelings.

Each session ended with a behavioral homework assignment. The assignment encouraged the parents to use some aspects of the new techniques at home. In addition, parents were encouraged to discuss these concepts with their spouse or the person with whom they lived. At the beginning of each session, parents were asked to share the experiences they had in using the techniques at home (Rickel & Dudley, 1983).

In general, the sessions were received very favorably by the parents, who indicated that they felt better about themselves as parents and were enjoying their children. The parents also reported feeling more confident about their ability to handle specific problem situations.

The effectiveness of the parent training program was evaluated with a treatment versus placebo control group format involving both center-city and suburban parents. The placebo control group programs consisted of the same number and length of sessions as those in the treatment programs and were nondirective discussions of the participants' parenting experience.

Prior to the program the center-city parents as a whole were more restrictive (i.e., expected conformity to demands) than were suburban parents as measured on the Rickel Modified Child Rearing Practices Report (Rickel & Biasatti, 1982). There was no preprogram difference between center-city parents and suburban parents on the nurturance dimension. From pre- to postprogram, experimentally trained parents decreased significantly on self-reports of restrictiveness. Furthermore, a significantly greater change was noted for center-city experimental parents trained in conjunction with the Preschool Project than for the suburban parents given the experimental training (Rickel, Dudley, & Berman, 1980).

The Detroit Parent Training Project has been adapted for implementation with teenage mothers. The longitudinal project, which began in 1986, provides a comprehensive 6-month program of parent education designed to enrich the adolescent mothers' knowledge of child development information, evaluate and enhance their parent-child interactions, and help them identify and manage stress more effectively. The goals are being achieved by conducting individual and small group training sessions with teenage mothers in order to disseminate information, discuss shared concerns, and promote social support networking. Participants have been recruited from Detroit City and Wayne County Public Schools Continuing Education Programs and are mothers of infants. These individuals were assigned to one of two groups: a training group and a control group. All groups received pre- and posttesting with parental attitude and personality measures. The effect of the parent training program was evaluated relative to the control group on maternal attitude and personality variables and on measures of infant development.

In addition to the focus on enhancing parent effectiveness, the Detroit Teen Parent Project is concerned with the development of an early identification model. The purpose of the model is twofold: (1) to identify personality and situational factors indicative of teen pregnancy and (2) given the occurrence of pregnancy, to identify personality, situational, and attitudinal factors associated with adaptive and maladaptive parenting styles. Such a model will provide mental health professionals with a useful tool for the identification of teenage girls at risk for early pregnancy and will provide a set of early indicators of future parenting problems.

CONTINUING EDUCATION FOR GIRLS

The inception of the Continuing Education for Girls Program in Michigan was a response by local school educators to the growing need created by the increasing numbers of school-age pregnancies. The CEG Program was designed to assist these girls in continuing their education, reduce the percentage of dropouts, and motivate their return to regular school. The perceived insensitivity, real or unreal, that the pregnant adolescent experiences in her regular school setting usually precipitates her seeking an alternative to meet her educational needs while pregnant.

The organization of the CEG Program is that of a secondary school for pregnant girls. It operates on the same schedule, within the guidelines, and under the regulation of the regular school programs. Girls in grades 7 through 12 attend classes that are in some instances multigraded (e.g., seventh and eighth grades combined) and flexible, with individualized instruction, group teaching, and team teaching. The service provisions include an educational component of daily instructional classes (i.e., courses in reading, math, social studies, communication, business/clerical) taught by certified teachers; health services that include counseling, referral and thorough follow-up for the delivery of medical assistance, and mental health support from a guidance counselor and parent specialist; and social services that focus on personal relationships, family problems, and the identification and use of community resources. Exploration of options and decision-making in the areas of child care, adoption arrangements, and family occur. The existence of a child care laboratory at the site allows for the safe care of the infants and an instructional opportunity for students to demonstrate parenting and care skills. Career training in the area of child care services is also facilitated through this laboratory environment.

The Detroit Teen Parent Project thus works in conjunction with CEG programs to reduce the negative outcomes of teenage pregnancy. Based on a peer advocate model of intervention, particular areas of interest were the effect of social supports on the new mother's effectiveness and satisfaction as a mother and the role of personality variables in the adolescent's parenting style. Presently in its third year of operation, findings from the project support prior research in the field and offer new insights.

PARTICIPANTS

One hundred twenty-four subjects were drawn from two alternative high schools expressly for pregnant or parenting teenage girls. One school is located in the center city and serves a mainly nonwhite population. The school provides medical care, counseling, nursery care, and parent skills training, in addition to a regular curriculum. The girls elect to attend the school and are allowed to remain enrolled through the year in which their babies are born. The second school serves a white population and differs in that the girls are allowed to remain until graduation if they choose. Day care is also provided for their children. All girls, from both schools, were between the ages of 14 and 19, the mean age being 16.1. Three fourths of the girls were pregnant or parenting for the first time. One fourth were pregnant for at least the second time.

QUESTIONNAIRES

Various forms of measurement were used in an interview to assess each adolescent mother's background, childrearing strategies, stress level, interpersonal support, and personality characteristics. The measures can be found in the Appendix, with the exception of the personality inventory. For the results presented in this chapter the demographic information will be utilized from the interview questionnaire (see Appendix, page 150) as well as the Rickel Modified Child Rearing Practices Report, the Perceived Social Support Network Inventory, the Mother's Opinion Measure, the Neonatal Perception Inventory, the Degree of Bother Inventory, and the Minnesota Multiphasic Personality Inventory.

The Rickel Modified Child Rearing Practices Report (R-CRPR) (Block, 1965; Rickel & Biasatti, 1982) is a questionnaire focusing on parental values and attitudes toward children (see Appendix, page 171). The subjects are asked to respond to 40 items using a Likert scale, with 1 meaning "not at all descriptive of me" and 7 meaning "highly descriptive of me." Factor analysis of this instrument has revealed that it measures two factors: restrictiveness (parental strictness and authoritarian style) and nurturance (parental givingness and supportive encouragement).

The factors have been found to have adequate internal reliability, with Cronbach's alphas of .85 for the Restrictiveness scale and .84 for the Nurturance scale in an undergraduate sample and .82 for both scales in a parent sample. Evidence for the construct validity of the R-CRPR is a study which revealed that parents with high Restrictiveness scores had children who were more likely to use evasion in solving parent-child problems, while parents with high Nurturance scores had children who were less likely to turn to authority figures to solve interpersonal problems (Jones, Rickel, & Smith, 1980).

The instrument used to measure the teens' interpersonal resources was the Perceived Social Support Network Inventory (Oritt, Paul, & Behrmann, 1985), which questions the subject about significant others in her life (see Appendix, page 169). The format includes a list of all the individuals who form the subject's social support network and classification of the type of support each individual offers—emotional, material, physical, and so forth. Since this instrument gave each teen the opportunity to self-report the people she would turn to in a time of stress, it reflects the amount of support that she perceives to be accessible to her.

The Mother's Opinion Measure (MOM), developed by the author for use in this study, is a 10-item questionnaire that requires the subject to state how she would respond to commonly encountered, stressful child management situations (see Appendix, page 164). Responses are recorded verbatim by interviewers and are then placed into classifications such as "spank" or "reason with the child," "meet the child's physical needs," "change personal plans," and so forth. Additionally, the teenagers are asked to suggest various toys that can be made at home, describe a typical day for their baby, plan a day's meals and snacks for a 1-year-old, and comment on the appropriateness of talking and/or reading to an infant.

Two factors or dimensions have been found to be measured by this instrument: (1) the use of behavior reinforcement in child management and (2) the mother's awareness of child development. Teens who score high on the behavior reinforcement dimension are likely to advocate using positive and negative reinforcement in managing their children, whereas girls who score low on this factor seldom report using behavior reinforcement techniques in their parenting repertoires. Additionally, girls who score high on the developmental enhancement dimension appear to have a basic knowledge of children's developmental stages as well as an awareness of how to enhance child development.

Modified versions of Broussard's Neonatal Perception Inventory II (NPI) and Degree of Bother Inventory (DBI) (see Appendix, pages 162 and 163) were used in our study to assess adolescent mothers' perceptions of their infants. Items for both instruments were selected by Broussard on the basis of her past clinical experience with young mothers' concerns about their babies. For instance, on the NPI the mother is asked "How much crying do you think the average baby does?" and then "How much crying does your infant do?" Broussard believes a mother's interactions with her newborn will be influenced by her perception of her or his behavior and appearance. Because of the great emphasis our culture places on being better than average, infants are considered to be at risk when their mothers do not rate them above average (Broussard and Hartner, 1971).

Similarly, on the DBI mothers are asked to indicate how much they have been bothered by their infant's crying, spitting up, sleeping patterns, and so forth. This instrument identifies those areas that constitute problem areas for the young mother with regard to typical infant behaviors.

The final instrument used was the Minnesota Multiphasic Personality Inventory (MMPI) (Hathaway, 1946), an objective technique of personality assessment whereby the respondent answers true or false to a series of questions. Only the first 366 items were used in the study, as many adolescents object to the length of the test and find the repetitive nature of the questions to be boring. A 366-item version provides the requisite number of items for all scales except the K scale (Defensiveness) and scale 0 (Social Introversion). The adolescents' MMPI profiles were not required to pass a validity check (evaluation of F-K scale differences) per the recommendations of Archer, White, and Orvin (1979) and Ehrenworth and

Archer (1985), who note that rigid validity criteria result in the exclusion of large numbers of adolescent profiles from analyses. The Social Introversion scale was not used in that it plays an insignificant role in the formation of two-point code types, which were used in the data analysis. Thus, it was felt that a 366-item MMPI would increase compliance without compromising the validity of the results. The mothers were instructed to answer all questions, if possible.

Adolescent norms (Archer, 1987) were used to interpret the personality profiles, and the mothers were placed into subgroups on the basis of their MMPI code type. The resulting subgroups were normal (all personality scales within normal limits), neurotic (self-absorbed girls exhibiting either high anxiety or depressive symptoms), characterological (somewhat rebellious teens who are likely to be nonconforming and resistant toward authority), socially alienated (socially withdrawn or isolated girls who are likely to be viewed by others as socially deviant in their thinking and/or actions), and unclassified (personality scales were elevated above normal for these girls, but their profiles did not fit into any of the existing categories).

A modified version of the PERI Life Events Scale (Dohwenrend & Dohwenrend, 1974) was also administered but not included in the results to date (see Appendix, page 174).

PROCEDURE

Each subject completed a personal, confidential interview with a trained interviewer. Research assistants were trained in interviewing techniques and in the use of the structured interview questionnaire through roleplaying and behavior rehearsal with faculty and upper-level graduate students also from Wayne State University. Administration of the structured interview required approximately 1 hour per subject. All items were read to the subjects to ensure adequate understanding. After the interview the girls completed the Minnesota Multiphasic Personality Inventory (MMPI) as a group. Subjects were encouraged to ask for clarification of items when necessary and were given a token gift for their babies who on average were three months of age when testing was completed.

DEMOGRAPHIC FACTORS IN TEENAGE PREGNANCY

A maritally disruptive household membership was experienced by 46% of the girls. Only 26% of the girls came from two-parent families, and 17% of the girls had mothers who never married, as can be seen in Table 1. The finding that only 26% of the girls have two parents in their homes is significant in light of the role that familial support is thought to play in the lives of young mothers. It suggests that the girls' families are themselves

Table 1   Demographics of Sample

	N	%
Race		
Black	69	55.6
White	55	44.4
Age		
14	7	5.6
15	23	18.5
16	22	17.7
17	22	17.7
18	13	10.5
19	1	.8
Number of times pregnant		
1	96	77.4
2	23	18.5
3	3	2.5
Parents marital status		
Married	32	25.8
Separated	20	16.1
Divorced	37	29.8
Never married	21	16.9
Career plans[a]		
Stay home with baby	49	28.3
Continue education	47	27.2
Trade school	11	6.4
College	33	19.1
Graduate school	4	2.3
Get a job	29	16.8

[a] Subjects could give two responses.

stressed by the personal and economic difficulties attendant upon many single-parent households and thus may or may not be able to provide effective social support to their daughters and grandchildren.

Ninety-three percent of the girls endorse a religious belief system (e.g., believing in God makes life meaningful and helps you become a stronger and better person). Fifty-two percent of these individuals attend church on a regular basis, with Catholic and Baptist being the religions most represented. The religious predominations in the sample may account for the lack of birth control methods used and why the girls elected to keep their babies.

More than 50% of the subjects reported an inability to maintain school performance during pregnancy. A common concern among the teen mothers was the conflict they felt between spending time with their babies in the evening and doing their homework. In addition, many of the girls we interviewed reported feeling exhausted much of the time due to their baby's erratic sleep patterns and feeding demands.

Fifty-five percent of the teens plan to continue their education, and over 30% plan to stay home after they have had their babies. Forty-three percent of the girls expressed a desire to pursue college and/or careers. However, research on these populations has shown that teen mothers often experience early truncation of their education, resulting in entry into the job market at the lower end, and in most instances not reaching their career potential.

The data revealed a profile of the adolescent mother. In general, 21% of the sample were pregnant for at least the second time, and of the total sample 31% did not use any form of contraception. Twenty-six percent of the adolescent females were happy about their pregnancy, and 59% were scared or confused. On the other hand, over 50% of the males fathering these babies, as reported by teen mothers, were happy to learn of the pregnancy. In addition, 85% of the girls reported that they had not planned their pregnancy.

The demographic findings in our sample support other research pointing to a general trend toward earlier and more teen pregnancies. The fact that one fifth of our sample, with a mean age of only 16, were experiencing a repeat pregnancy clearly shows the need for earlier educational intervention at the preteen level for both boys and girls than is presently available.

PERSONALITY TYPES AND PARENTING STYLES

Depression

In assessing the relationship between the maternal variables of nurturance and restrictiveness and dimensions of personality as measured by the MMPI, a significantly negative relationship was found between nurturance and depression. This indicates that the more depressed the girls reported feeling, the fewer nurturant attitudes they endorsed. High scores on the nurturance factor reflect a flexible parenting style characterized by respect for the child's feelings.

Our results yield several clues to factors that promote nurturant behavior in young mothers and also to those factors that inhibit or prevent it. The negative relationship between depression and nurturance suggests that teen mothers experiencing depression may be unable to extend care to their children, as part of an overall impairment in functioning. It is intuitively plausible that social withdrawal, uncertainty, and poor self-care would all be behavioral concomitants of depression and thus would also be negatively related to nurturance. These and perhaps other depressive symptoms may serve as behavioral signals that could alert health care providers and other professionals to the need for mental health intervention for these mothers and their babies. Such early intervention could help prevent the establishment of a pattern of poor mother-child interaction.

Rebelliousness

A significantly negative relationship was also found between restrictiveness and rebelliousness as well as nontraditional role orientation. Thus, girls who themselves resisted authority were less likely to state that they would seek to control their child's behavior and feelings. Further, girls who shunned traditional women's roles were far less restrictive in their reported parenting styles than teens with a traditional role orientation. High scores on the restrictiveness factor reflect the controlling, authoritarian aspects of childrearing.

MMPI SUBGROUPS AND PARENTING ATTITUDES

Overall the MMPI results indicated that by using adolescent norms and a clinical cutoff score of 65T only 20% of the sample fell within the normal limits of psychological adjustment. Approximately 18% of the girls were classified as neurotic, 22% as characterological, and 20% as socially alienated.

These results were somewhat surprising. Though personality research with teenage samples has yielded mixed results in the past, most recently pregnant and/or parenting teens have not been viewed as a pathological group (e.g., Barth et al., 1983; Ralph et al., 1984). The fact that only one fifth of the sample fell within normal adjustment limits on the MMPI implies that a need exists for preventive interventions. It is unclear, however, whether these adolescents were disturbed prior to pregnancy or whether the realistic demands of parenthood were causing immediate tribulation.

To further delineate the role of personality in parental attitudes and values, the girls were placed into subgroups on the basis of their MMPI profiles. An analysis was performed to determine whether the groups differed in their self-reported attitudes of nurturance and restrictiveness.

Nurturance

With respect to nurturance, it was found that the neurotic and characterological groups differed significantly from one another (see Fig. 1). Girls in the neurotic group reported far fewer nurturant attitudes than did their peers in the characterological group.

Group differences on measures of nurturance and restrictiveness suggest that self-absorbed girls whose profiles are in the neurotic group are doing relatively little parenting. A modest correlation between nurturance and restrictiveness ($r = .32$, $p < .01$) implies that without order and a sense of control there may be little mutual respect between parent and child. The fact that girls in the neurotic subgroup are low on both nurturant and restrictive attitudes suggests a low level of involvement with their offspring.

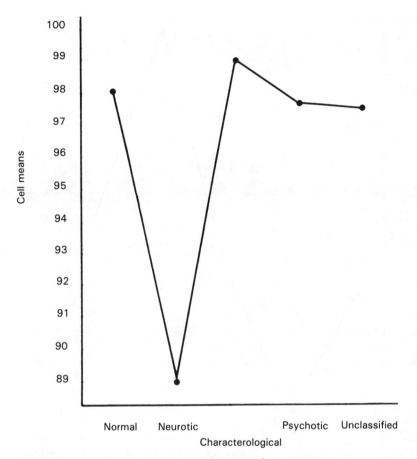

Cell means

Normal   Neurotic   Psychotic   Unclassified
                    Characterological

Figure 1   Plot of cell means for personality groups for nurturance.

Restrictiveness

For restrictiveness the girls whose MMPI profiles were in the socially alienated subgroup differed significantly from the girls in the neurotic subgroup,
with the socially alienated subgroup being more restrictive (see Fig. 2)
(Thomas, 1988). This high level of restrictiveness for socially alienated
mothers is of interest. The adolescent profile of the socially alienated teen,
as described by Archer (1987), is characterized by social isolation and
withdrawal; reluctance to engage in interpersonal relationships; and nonconforming, unconventional, socially deviant attitudes. In our sample this
subgroup was made up of largely nonwhite, center-city teens from Baptist
backgrounds. Their strict, traditional childrearing attitudes may be a product of religious teaching, and their feelings of alienation may be related to

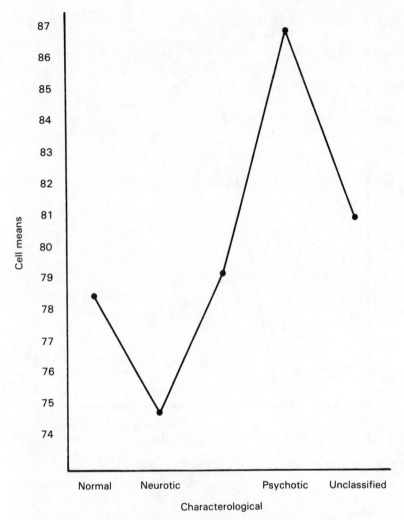

Figure 2   Plot of cell means for personality groups for restrictiveness.

the difficulties many minorities face living in predominantly white, middle-class society.

Though it is unclear whether girls in the socially alienated subgroup are truly exhibiting "pathology" or whether they are merely responding to feelings of isolation, their highly restrictive parenting styles are of concern. In their 1980 study, Jones et al. found that children whose parents espoused restrictive parenting values had poorer problem-solving skills than children whose parents were more nurturant. It would appear, therefore, that intervention methods to enhance nurturance and more flexible parenting attitudes in these mothers would aid teens' offspring in developing social problem-solving tactics and personal coping strategies (Webster-Stratton, 1987).

Observations of the girls' behavior supported these findings in that a positive relationship was found between nurturance and subjects appearing self-assured or well groomed. Further, there was a negative relationship between restrictiveness and observations of apprehension. Thus, it appears that girls who were uncertain or apprehensive at the time of the interview (often falling within the neurotic category) scored low on both nurturance and restrictiveness.

SOCIAL SUPPORT AND PARENTING STYLE

Turning to issues of social support, a significantly positive relationship was found between nurturance and the extent of the social support network as well as the number of family supports. Restrictiveness was negatively correlated with the perceived satisfaction of the support network, especially that received from friends. However, the presence of a boyfriend in the social support network had a negative relationship with all other sources of social support. In addition, the results showed that satisfaction with support provided by a boyfriend was negatively related to mothers' satisfaction with the baby (Butler, 1989).

The number of people offering social support to the mother appears to be a major factor in the presence of nurturant behavior. Social support is known to buffer the effects of stress and to ameliorate depression. It may be that the relationship between social support and nurturance stems from the fact that support promotes more nurturant parenting styles. In any case the present results suggest that a brief social network survey might be an effective device for targeting teen mothers in need of special assistance. It further suggests that interventions targeted toward helping teen mothers establish and maintain social support contacts may be beneficial in terms of improving the mothers' ability to care for their children (Atlas & Rickel, 1988; de Anda, 1984; Stevens, 1988).

Teen mothers' boyfriends play a significant role in shaping the girls' social networks and may affect their interactions with their children. The finding that teen mothers who maintain contact with boyfriends tend to have less contact with family, friends, and virtually all other supports is alarming for several reasons. Such dependence on a single source of support, which is not likely to be stable over time, builds a high level of insecurity into the lives of both mother and baby. The paucity of other support also means that the young mother lacks role models, a peer group with which to identify, and simple material assistance in everyday tasks of living. A teen who must shoulder so many psychological and material burdens will have difficulty being an effective parent. Social isolation of young couples is a known risk factor for serious family dysfunction.

Finally, our results indicate that satisfaction with support provided by a boyfriend is negatively related to the young mother's satisfaction with her baby. The role of the fathers in interacting with the babies is open to question. These findings have implications for community-based interventions in that, for this population, community outreach involving the young men may be an effective means of dealing with the incipient problems of this group. Since they are unlikely to approach sources of help themselves, peer advocates through school and church agencies might be more effective than hospital-based parent groups.

PREDICTORS OF PARENTING STYLE

To further delineate the origins of parenting styles among teenage mothers, several variables were put into a prediction equation in an effort to predict parenting style. Among the independent variables were social support, religion, the adolescent's awareness of developmental enhancement, and her self-reported agreement with using positive and negative reinforcement as a child management strategy. The canonical correlation analysis was successful in predicting nurturant or restrictive parenting styles (Wilks = 3.18, $p < .01$).

To more fully understand the relationships among variables, regression analyses were employed using nurturance and restrictiveness as dependent variables. It appears that the best overall predictor of nurturing parental values in this analysis was the subject's religion. In our sample the adolescents coming from more fundamental protestant backgrounds (e.g., Baptist, Jehovah Witness) were less likely to espouse nurturant parenting attitudes than girls from Catholic or other protestant religions. It should be noted, however, that there were significant racial differences within religious groups, with blacks being more often involved in Baptist or fundamental Christian movements and whites preferring Catholic or other protestant religions (e.g., Presbyterian, Lutheran). Thus, it may be that differences in parenting values reflect broader cultural or racial values rather than religious orientation (Rickel, Williams, & Loigman, 1988). Interestingly, adolescents from fundamentalist Christian religions appeared to have less extensive social support systems than did girls from Catholic or other protestant religions.

For the parenting style of restrictiveness, two variables appeared to be significant predictors: (1) the preferred use of behavior reinforcement in child management and (2) the extensiveness of the social support network. Both of these variables were negatively associated with restrictiveness. This suggests that girls who rely on behavior reinforcement as a principal means of child management and who have broader support networks are likely to score low on restrictiveness items and higher on nurturance items.

The high levels of church attendance and religious beliefs among the adolescents in our sample raise possibilities for future intervention strategies. Churches are a traditional social focus and could be effective vehicles for community-level intervention. Such a focus might have the beneficial effect of strengthening connections among already existing sources of support. In addition, this would be an effective way to package educational efforts in a way that is sensitive to local culture and acceptable to the recipients of intervention (Rickel, Gerrard, & Iscoe, 1984).

MATERNAL SATISFACTION AMONG ADOLESCENTS

Because maternal satisfaction is intuitively related to the nurturing behaviors of mothers in general, an analysis was undertaken to look at factors relating to adolescents' satisfaction with their offspring and the amount of bother they perceive their babies to be. Naturally, only those teens in the study who had already had their babies were used in the analysis ($N = 62$).

Several variables were investigated as predictors of satisfaction: the teen's reaction to news of her pregnancy, the availability and extensiveness of social support, complications during delivery, whether or not the infant was full term, and the presence or absence of physical abnormalities at birth.

Several interesting relationships emerged among the prenatal care and outcome variables (see Table 2—note: the variable of Prenatal Checkups was reverse scored). For instance, whether or not the baby was carried to term was significantly correlated with both birth complications and physical abnormalities of the child. In addition, the more favorably the pregnancy was received by the mother and her boyfriend the more prenatal checkups the mother reported. The number of prenatal visits was in turn related to

Table 2 Correlations among Variables

	Complications	Prematurity	Physical abnormalities	Prenatal check-ups	Pregnancy problems
Complications	1.0	.57[a]	.47[a]	− .05	.21[b]
Prematurity	.57[a]	1.0	.85[a]	− .20	.01
Physical abnormalities	.47[a]	.85[a]	1.0	− .18	− .06
Prenatal checkups	− .05	− .20	− .18	1.0	.33[a]
Pregnancy problems	.21[b]	.01	− .06	.33[a]	1.0

[a] $p < .01$.
[b] $p < .05$.

the number of problems encountered during pregnancy; thus, the more frequently the teen saw a medical professional the fewer health problems she reported. Further, a higher number of problems during pregnancy was associated with birth complications. These findings support the need for quality, affordable prenatal care for adolescent mothers.

Alcohol and the use of over-the-counter drugs during pregnancy were also found to be related. Of interest is the fact that girls who reported taking over-the-counter medicines also had fewer prenatal checkups than teens who had not. It is typically recommended that a pregnant woman not use any medication due to the possible negative effects on the developing fetus. Perhaps teenagers who do not initiate early and regular prenatal care are not aware of the need to abstain from such substances.

The use of alcohol during pregnancy was also related to the mother being less happy about the initial news of her pregnancy. Possibly the mother drank as a solace to the depression she felt about being pregnant or perhaps use of alcohol was related to her original conception. In chapter 1 alcohol use was listed as a variable predisposing young women to having unplanned intercourse without taking contraceptive precautions. Interestingly, neither alcohol nor tobacco use was related to any of the negative outcome measures utilized (i.e., birth complications, physical abnormalities of the newborn, or prematurity). Use of illegal drugs was not used as a variable because none of the girls reported having used any during their pregnancy. It should be noted that this is highly unlikely given the diverse sample from which these mothers was drawn. What is more plausible is that the young mothers were not answering honestly, perhaps because they feared a breech of confidentiality.

A canonical correlation analysis was employed using the independent variables listed above and the Modified Neonatal Perception Inventory as the dependent variable. Overall the variables were successful in predicting mothers' satisfaction with their offspring (Wilks $= 10.76$, $p < .01$). In particular, it was found that positive perceptions of one's baby were negatively related to both complications during delivery and the presence of physical abnormalities. When complications and physical abnormalities were absent, mothers held positive perceptions about their babies (e.g., perceiving their child as either average or above average). Conversely, when complications or abnormalities were present at birth, teen mothers were likely to perceive their infants more negatively.

For an index of perceived degree of bother caused by their infant, whether or not the child was carried to term was the best predictor. Adolescents who gave birth to premature, low-birth-weight infants were likely to report infant care as being more bothersome than girls whose babies were full term. The long-term impact of prematurity on mother and infant has been discussed at length in chapter 3, where low birth weight, prematurity, and congenital defects were listed as possible precursors of child abuse and maltreatment. It would seem that increased efforts to ameliorate attendant birth difficulties in this young population would have multiple benefits. Enhancing adolescent mothers' social support networks while providing easy-access quality prenatal care may aid in diminishing negative outcomes for teenagers and their offspring (Atkinson & Rickel, 1984).

CONCLUSION

We have examined some of the risk factors in teen mothers' social environments and have suggested directions for program planning and intervention. Our Detroit Teen Parent Project is in the process of implementing several of these suggested directions for program development and intervention. The Project, which utilizes peer counselors who are closely matched to the young mothers, is designed to enhance parenting competencies and reduce the incidence of unplanned repeat pregnancies. Outcome evaluation and longitudinal study of the impact of these school and community-level interventions are anticipated and will yield additional insights into the development of maternal competence and children's health and well-being.

Chapter 5

The Intervention Program

The Detroit Teen Parent Project based at Wayne State University has two purposes. One is to investigate the social and psychological variables associated with becoming pregnant while an adolescent and how those variables affect the teen mother's childrearing abilities and practices. The other is to offer social support, help, and guidance to young mothers through a one-on-one intervention with trained peer advocates.

A group of Wayne State University undergraduates volunteered, in exchange for course credit, to act as peer advocates for an academic year. The rationale for this intervention is the finding that too often teen mothers are without sufficient social support. Indeed, they often become pregnant in response to family troubles, loneliness, low self-esteem, and a need to be popular among peers. Once the baby is born, there may be even less support and friendly contact available, particularly outside the family. Girls may not feel at home among other mothers who are twice their age, and peer contacts may dwindle as parenting responsibilities increase. Yet such contacts and support can provide a needed buffer against stress as well as a source of sound factual information and advice on coping with the demands of parenthood.

Research suggests that both the stress-buffering and the parent training aspects of social support may help prevent or reduce maternal distress and child neglect and abuse. The case study method serves as an important part of the research design. Yin (1984) details the proper application of different research strategies according to the research question under consideration and the circumstances in which the research is conducted. Commonly, the survey method has been used to gather descriptions of existing phenomena, answering the "who, what, where, how many, and how much" questions. These instruments yield correlational, not causal, data. "How" and "why" questions have traditionally been the province of the experimental method. The latter, however, presupposes control over surrounding events and conditions. In much of modern social science research, experimental control is either impossible or undesirable. When the subjects of interest are the naturally occurring interactions of people in a given environmental context, experimental manipulation would destroy the object of study. According to Yin, when the task is to discover the "how" and "why" of a behavioral event through naturalistic observation, case study is the method of choice.

The course of the intervention is thus presented in descriptive form, as a series of excerpts from journals written by the volunteer peer advocates. The intervention itself consists of two individuals in an interpersonal relationship; therefore, its effectiveness lies more in process than in content. Each intervention plan was unique to the specific needs of the adolescent mother and often changed in response to the progress of the dyadic relationship. Excerpts from the journals of several peer advocates have been juxtaposed to present a composite picture of the intervention experience.

THE PEER ADVOCATES

All peer advocates were members of an undergraduate Field Study course in psychology offered by Wayne State University. Prerequisites for this course included Introductory Psychology, Developmental Psychology, and Abnormal Psychology. Students registering for Field Study could choose to work in a community agency offering psychological services to a variety of populations or to become a peer advocate in the Teen Parent Project. All students were required to make a 1-year commitment to the agency or project of their choice, for which they received 3 hours of credit per semester. Students were not allowed to receive a salary for their contributions (6 to 10 hours of work per week). Field study is recommended to undergraduate students as a means of obtaining hands on experience in the field of psychology, which may ultimately aid them is securing a job or gaining admission to a graduate program.

Those choosing involvement in the Teen Parent Project were screened by the project staff to ensure their suitability for the project. Important considerations were the advocate's apparent reliability, emotional stability, and interest and concern regarding adolescent parenting. Further, each advocate was required to have adequate means of transportation.

The student advocates have typically been a diverse population. Each year the proportion of black and white advocates has been about equal, although the vast majority of "little sisters" from the continuing education facility utilized in the study have been black. The school's administrator believes that racial diversity of the advocates is an important aspect of exposing the young mothers to a broad range of social experiences and values.

Most of the advocates have been in their late teens or early 20s and living at home with their parents while completing the latter stages of their undergraduate educations. In addition, most advocates have held jobs outside the university and as such were required to juggle a number of responsibilities while acting as peer advocates. Socioeconomic status of the peer advocates has varied and appears to be representative of the overall student population at Wayne State University. A small percentage of the advocates have been married, and each year there is typically one advocate who was herself a teenage parent.

Peer advocates were expected to have two "little sisters" and to spend about 3 hours per week with each of them. How they spent that time was to be agreed on by the advocates and their girls. Going to movies and fast food restaurants were among the favorite activities of the young mothers, and reimbursement of expenses was provided for the advocates. Additionally, each advocate was asked to keep a journal recording weekly activities as well as exploring his or her feelings about the advocate relationship.

As previously described, an alternative school for pregnant teens in center-city Detroit was the intervention site. The school is part of the Detroit public school system, but attendance there is strictly voluntary; the girls must request to be transferred there. Most are day students, but there is a dormitory that houses about 20 girls who either are wards of the court or simply have no homes. Medical care and an infant nursery are available. A regular academic program is supplemented with remedial tutoring when needed. Special classes in child care procedures are also part of the program. The girls may stay only until the end of the school year in which the baby is born; after that, they must return to regular schools.

The principal of the Booth School compiled a list of the girls who appeared to be in greatest need. While most of the young mothers could benefit from having a peer advocate, some were more at risk than others (e.g., poor school attendance, chaotic family structure, and few personal or economic resources). The principal then interviewed each of our volunteer advocates in an effort to carefully match each girl with a compatible advocate. When a girl had a special interest, for example, wanting to start her own business, an advocate was chosen who had similar interests or actual experience in that area. The initial meetings between the girls and their advocates, whom they immediately dubbed "our big sisters," were characterized by mingled shyness and eagerness on both sides.

Entries from the journals of two peer advocates describe their first impressions:

> Today is our field study meeting. We went to the director of the school. It surprised me to find out that many of the girls that she works with there either get pregnant on purpose, or aren't very surprised or upset that they are. These girls are falling for the line that "if you love me, you'll have my baby." It amazes me that they would believe it. It just emphasizes what a different "culture" they live in. It was weird, too, that at 21, I felt old. I felt that already I had had more experiences and more opportunities than they will ever have. I couldn't imagine having a baby now, much less a school age child, which is what some of these girls will have when they are 21.

> *October 27*

> I had my interview with Ms. Andrews today at 1:30 p.m. The focus of the interview was how did I really feel about the issue of teen pregnancy and girls who become pregnant. Mrs. Andrews wanted my prejudices or biased opinions as well as any previous positive feedback I had received, as well as any personal experiences with teen pregnancy I may have had. At first I felt the interview was more of an interrogation, but at the same time I realized Ms. Andrews had to get some idea of the character of the unknown individual the school was involving with one of their students. I assume I handled the interview to her satisfaction, because I was allowed to meet my "sister" at the end of the interview. We were given five minutes to exchange phone numbers and get a general feel or idea of what the intervention would involve.

> My "sister's" name is Jody S., she is eighteen years old, and her baby is six months old. Jody expresses herself clearly and freely, and was openly grateful to have somebody care about her from the community beyond the school or her immediate family. She wondered why another girl with more pressing problems had not been given the opportunity to gain some other coping skills and an increased awareness of other options life has to offer. I explained that the teachers at Booth School and Ms. Andrews had defined the criteria for the selection of the students who would receive big sisters, and they felt she would benefit from this experience. Ms. Andrews explained that Jody needed support in clarifying her career goals and also some additional information concerning the other options available in the area of continuing her education.

> My feelings from this first meeting are mixed. Jody comes from a family

where there is a strong religious persuasion. I feel I must be sensitive to Jody's beliefs and I will need to find out where she falls on the spectrum of the religion. The interview should give me a better insight into the question. I like Jody's attitude of expecting something rewarding to come from our exchange together.

November 14

The party at school gave me the opportunity to see a few of the other "sisters" involved in the research project. It was very enlightening to be greeted at the door by two eager faces inquiring as to whether or not I was going to be a "big sister." The thought brought back memories of growing up with my big sister at home and how today we are even closer as I grow a little older and a little wiser. I realize how important my sister has been at various transition periods in my life, and I know how valuable these kinds of exchanges can be in our lives. So I am truly grateful for this intervention experience.

TRAINING AND SUPERVISION OF THE ADVOCATES

Once the advocates had been approved for involvement with the project the task of training began. The questionnaire was introduced (see Appendix), and students were asked to study it carefully at home, generating any questions they might have about the appropriate procedures. During a designated class period questions were addressed, and the advocates role played an actual interview. This exercise had a twofold purpose, exposing any confusion the advocates might have with the interview process itself and giving further insight into how the advocates might deal with some of the sensitive issues relating to teenage pregnancy. Additionally, the advocates were instructed in the administration of the MMPI. Both the MMPI and the interview were to be completed prior to the advocate-mother dyads beginning a formal relationship with one another.

Training and supervision continued on a weekly basis as the advocates began meeting with their girls. The initial thrust of the intervention was social in nature, with the goal being the establishment of a trusting, caring relationship with their assigned young mothers. Advocates were encouraged to bring problems and concerns to the meeting for group discussion. Occasionally problems would arise during the week, and each advocate has an assigned staff member whom they could call when difficulties arose that they did not feel could wait until the meeting.

When rapport was established between the advocates and girls, other phases of the intervention were introduced, such as development of social resources, contraception, career-building, goal-setting, child development, and parenting issues. Speakers were brought in with the purpose of augmenting the curriculum. At each point, information was presented to the advocates, who in turn disseminated it to their assigned mothers.

At the end of the school year, the advocates were asked to compose an informal case study of their girls, which would include information as to the teen's developmental milestones, family structure, present life situation, and specific goals and plans. The teen mothers in our intervention program were mainly poor center-city blacks. Nearly all came from single-parent homes. Many received little support from their families, and some coped with problems that our volunteers had never even imagined. The following example is a case description written by Glenda's peer advocate:

CASE STUDY: GLENDA

Physical Description

Glenda is short, a little chubby, with large dark eyes. She gives the impression of a young child-like girl, with her round face and awkward carriage. Her pregnancy gives her a strange, incongruous look of adulthood, as though she were dressed in an older woman's clothes. Her guarded look alone belies her youth.

Family Structure

Glenda, 16 years old, is currently living with her parents, a sister and a brother. Her sister is 14 years old and her brother is nine years old. She gets along with both siblings. She and her parents are getting along now as compared to their relationship before.

Developmental Milestones

There are no important events that happened to Glenda during her preschool and childhood years that she can recall. Her most vivid memories are those of her teen years. When she was fourteen years old she ran away from home because she was very unhappy, and she wasn't getting along with her parents. When her mother couldn't control her, she put Glenda into a girls' home. After a few months Glenda ran away from there and went back home. For a while everything was going fine, then Glenda got pregnant. When she found out that she was pregnant she was scared to tell her mother and father. She couldn't believe that it could happen to her, and waited a couple of months before telling her parents. That pregnancy ended in miscarriage. After the miscarriage, Glenda was depressed and couldn't accept what had happened. She started seeing a psychiatrist, because she thought that she was going crazy and she didn't have anyone to talk to. She felt so alone and empty that she just needed someone to talk to about her problems. She couldn't handle the pressure of the loss of her baby, so she ran away from home again. At this time she started seeing a boy named Jeff, and she went to live with him and his mother, without her parents' knowledge.

Glenda lived with them for a year. During this time she quit school and stayed home every day. She wasn't happy at Jeff's house either, but she didn't want to go back home. Jeff's mother is a drug addict and her son dealt in drugs. Glenda remembers an event which happened while she was living with them. She was taken as a hostage because Jeff's mother stole money from a drug deal. Two men broke into the house, and pulled a gun on Jeff and Glenda. The ordeal lasted for two days. The men held a gun to Glenda's head and ordered Jeff to find his mother with the money or they'd kill Glenda. After a couple of days the mother was found and the money was given to the men. They left after they got their money. After this incident, Glenda and Jeff left his mother's house. Jeff went to live with his father and step-mother, and Glenda went back home with her parents.

After things settled down she found herself pregnant for the second time. When Glenda and Jeff had been living with his mother they both wanted a baby, and he was trying to get her pregnant. She wasn't using any type of birth control at this time, but despite many tries they were unsuccessful. Glenda thought that maybe something was wrong with her physically. She went to see a gynecologist for a checkup but the doctor found nothing wrong with her. After many more unsuccessful tries, they found out that the problem was with Jeff. The doctor told them that his sperm wasn't potent enough because of previous drug and alcohol abuse. The doctor gave Jeff some vitamins to take and eventually Glenda got pregnant. When she found out she was really happy but Jeff got mad at her because he had changed his mind about having a baby. She was also afraid that this pregnancy might end in a miscarriage like the previous one. Fortunately, there were no complications. During this pregnancy Glenda was a ward of the court and was living with a foster family. She began attending Booth School when she was 7 months pregnant. Her family situation was still strained. Her natural mother came to see her at Booth on a regular basis, and wanted her to come back home. After long discussions between mother and daughter, Glenda decided to go back home and try to get along with her parents. At this time she has been getting along with her parents with no thoughts of running away from home again. Her parents are also helping her with the baby financially. Her main support network includes her mother and father. She now realized that her mother is very important to her and she had taken her for granted.

Glenda's parents didn't set an age when she could start dating. She had known Jeff ever since she was 12 years old, and they had been going out since then. After a couple of years Jeff and his family moved, but the two still kept in touch. Recently, Glenda broke up with Jeff because he wasn't treating her well. He doesn't support the baby and doesn't visit her. When Glenda was in the hospital having her baby, Jeff didn't come to see her or call her. She wants to file for child support so that he will help financially, but Glenda's mother doesn't believe in making a man pay if he doesn't want to. Her parents have told her that they'll help her as long as she needs it.

Present Life Situation

Glenda is finding it hard to care for the baby and attend school at the same time. She finds little time for herself and for friends. Her days are mainly composed of caring for the baby and doing her homework. She says that the baby keeps her up all night and it's hard to get up in the morning to get ready for school. Everyday she thanks God for her mom's understanding and support. Their relationship is fine and they are helping one another to make up for all the pain they've caused one another. Glenda knows that everything will be alright if she sticks with it and does not give up.

Specific Goals and Plans

As of now Glenda's priority is to finish High School and get her diploma because she is a year behind. She doesn't know if she is going to college but she knows that she'll try to give her daughter everything she can. She is planning to find a job and starting a college fund for her daughter because she doesn't want her to be a dropout like her parents. She isn't thinking about marriage, because she knows that she's too young and still immature in some ways. She is also aware that girls her age don't have the same responsibilities as she does and her priorities are different now that she has a baby.

Another case study further reveals serious family disturbance.

CASE STUDY: DARLENE

Physical Description

Darlene is a tall, slender girl with deeply set sad eyes. She is neatly dressed, well groomed and because of her height appears much older than her fifteen years.

Family Structure

For the past 15 years, Darlene has been living with her grandmother and step-grandfather. Her parents are separated, her father is in jail and her mother is currently living with a boyfriend. She has two brothers, 19 and 18 years old, and a step-sister who is 4 years old. I will now discuss Darlene's relationship with each of her family members.

Grandmother. Darlene's grandmother is her sole support. She has lived with her grandparents since she was a year old. Her grandmother is a cocktail waitress and the main breadwinner in the family. Darlene and her grandmother depend on each other more now as compared to before. There was a time when Darlene's grandmother couldn't control her behavior. She was in constant trouble in school as well as at home. She is now realizing that her grandmother is really important to her and that she can depend on her. Their relationship is fine, but Darlene can't talk to her about some things, such as boys and sex. Darlene doesn't think her grandmother really wants to know what she does when she isn't home.

Step-Grandfather. Darlene resents her grandfather because he is unemployed and doesn't help around the house. He takes advantage of her grandmother, by depending on her for financial support. He is always at home, the only time he leaves the house is when he and his friends go to the bars. He usually comes home drunk and stumbles all over the house. Then, he starts yelling at everyone in the house when he doesn't get his way. Darlene told me that this happens almost every night. She doesn't know what to do or say, she just wants her grandmother to throw her grandfather out. The grandparents are constantly arguing in front of the children.

Father. I've never met Darlene's father. She doesn't talk about him at all, and the only thing I know is that he is in jail.

Mother. I've met her mother once, when I came to pick Darlene up. Her mother isn't around much and Darlene feels that her mother doesn't care about any of them because she is never around much. Darlene doesn't know her mother well enough to consider her a mother. She recalls something that happened one time, one day she came home from school and found her mother in bed with someone. The mother saw her in the room but didn't acknowledge her and continued what they were doing. Her mother didn't take care of any of her children, instead she just dropped them off at grandma's.

Brothers. Both of her brothers live upstairs in the house. She feels closer to her older brother, David, than to her younger brother. When she needs advice or help with anything she goes to David. Both her brothers' girlfriends are pregnant.

Sister. Denise is 4 years old. Darlene doesn't like Denise because she thinks that she is a brat. She has to watch her sister all the time which leaves little time for Darlene to enjoy herself. I've told her that her sister just wants to play with someone and she shouldn't treat her like that. No one in the family spends any time with Denise, and she just needs a little attention.

Developmental Milestones

Darlene doesn't recall anything from her childhood, only that her mother wasn't around while she was growing up. Her grandmother raised her and her brothers.

When she was in junior high she was expelled from school for rowdy behavior. She usually got into fights and arguments with other girls in school. Last year she ran away from home and stayed with a friend of hers. She doesn't remember much about her father, he went to jail when she was still small and she doesn't talk much about him. She spent some time in a reform school, because the teachers, her mother, and grandmother couldn't control her. After spending some time in the reform school her behavior became worse, and she ran away from home again and was gone for a year. Her grandmother had no knowledge of her whereabouts. After a while she went back home to live with her grandparents.

After a few months, she met Ken (her boyfriend) and it was at this time that her behavior began to change. She told me that she changed because of Ken, she wanted to dress and act like a girl instead of a tomboy.

She met Ken when she was 14 years old, he was 17. She started dating when she was 14. Her grandmother didn't really set an age when she could start dating, nor did she have a curfew. Darlene and Ken started engaging in sex after they knew each other for a short time. She was not using any type of birth control, nor was he. When she found out that she was pregnant she was so scared she couldn't tell anyone because she was afraid that her grandmother might find out. Eventually, her grandmother found out and was so disappointed in Darlene. When Ken found out that Darlene was pregnant he was mad and told her that it wasn't his baby. After a while he finally accepted the fact that it was his baby, and both accepted what had happened and knew they had to make some plans. She decided to keep the baby and Ken will help financially.

Ken is 18 years old and currently attends Wayne State University. He is undecided about a major, and wants to quit school. His mother pays for his tuition and he is unemployed at the moment. He visits Darlene and the baby on a regular basis and is helping her financially.

Present Life Situation

Darlene had Ken Jr. on March 19, 1987. He weighed 6 pounds, 10 ounces. She was in labor for 12 hours, and she was in so much pain that she doesn't want to have another baby. She won't be able to go back to school until the end of April. She misses not being able to go back to school because she is bored at home.

Her grandmother helps her with the baby. Her biggest complaint is that she doesn't go out with her friends anymore, and is always at home with the baby. She knows that she has a lot of responsibilities and she has to sacrifice the fun she used to have.

Specific Goals and Plans

She wants to finish high school and later on go to college. I'm glad that she is thinking about furthering her education. She wants to be able to give her baby everything she can. She is determined to give her baby things that she never had. Ken has asked her to marry him but she said no. She knows that they are both too young to get married and being married may bring them more problems. She is satisfied with her present life and even though Ken Jr. was a mistake she is glad she had him.

In some cases the young mother has no family support at all. In fact, the families can even be a threat to the teenager's well-being. The following is a description of a young ward of the court whose child also was born into court custody.

CASE STUDY: AMY

On March 10, 1987, Amy gave birth to her first child. The fifteen year old mother experienced a long painful labor and sustained a third degree episiotomy. On Friday, March 6, she had been admitted to Grace Hospital. She suffered through three days of induced labor without dilating until her release on Sunday. On the following Tuesday Amy was re-admitted at 7:00 am and delivered her son at 4:55 pm. He weighed six pounds and one ounce and was a very healthy newborn. Although Amy wanted a girl she loved him instantly.

Family Structure

Amy's mother is not quite a perfect role model. She has three children and has never been married. Amy is the oldest, followed by Tommy 14, and Bill 13. Amy and Bill share the same biological parents but Tommy is only their half-brother. This arrangement doesn't seem to be detrimental to their relationship. They consider themselves siblings without reference to being "half" related. All three currently are in foster homes as wards of the court. Amy's mother was charged with neglect and abuse, a condition brought on by a drug dependency. The boys have been kept together, and Amy has talked to them but has only seen them a few times. Though she doesn't seem upset about not seeing her brothers, she misses her mother. Amy loves her mother deeply no matter what she does. Amy's father is in jail at present for robbery. She keeps a written correspondence with him, and he is furious with Amy's mother for losing custody of the kids again and has threatened her. Amy remembers her father being in and out of jail all her life and considers him an evil man. She even warns her mother to stay away from him when he is released. Though her view of her father is negative she confesses she still loves him too. Her family ties are very strong and she looks forward to her weekend visits to see them. Amy never plans to live with either of her parents again but she loves both almost out of duty. She has separated their wrong deeds from the persons. She forgives her mother for the lack of caring she shows and remembers the times when her mother wasn't on drugs. According to Amy the good times still outweigh the bad.

Developmental Milestones

This is not the first time Amy has been in a foster home. Five years ago her mother was heavily into drugs and the children were placed in the court's custody for six months. As I mentioned before, her father has not been a major influence in her life. Amy's models have been women and she relates better to women than men. Her grandmother and Aunt Debra have been important besides her mother. Amy and her family moved in with her grandma almost two years ago. It was then that Amy was just friends with Lee, then he started to say he loved her. When Amy approached her mother about getting some birth control her mother told her she wasn't old enough. Because Amy thought she loved Lee too she agreed to start a sexual relationship with him. They were in this relationship for a few months before Amy became pregnant. The week after she conceived, she and her brothers were put into foster care. When Amy told Lee she was carrying his child he denied that he was the father. Because Amy threatened to have blood tests taken, Lee admitted he was the father. Amy lived with her Aunt Debra until school started, and then she moved to the dorm at Booth. Lee was the first, and so far the only boy Amy has had intercourse with. Her family accepted her pregnancy because several relatives have had children out of wedlock. Her mother wasn't really happy but Amy looks at it as a chance to get out of the bad environment she lived in. Her mother never pushed school so she skipped a lot, which is why she is only in the 7th grade and not the 9th grade. Also, drugs have filled her surroundings and she doesn't want them as her life style.

Present Life Situation

Amy lives in a temporary foster home with her baby. She will be moved to a permanent home in a few months. She complains about her foster mother but when asked if she wants to leave she says everything is fine. The reason for this is because this foster home is close to her mother's house. She tries to make the best of the situation because she is afraid she will be moved to a home further away. Her Aunt Debra's house had been approved by the social worker as a place to visit, something she likes to do more often than her foster mother likes.

Amy handles the baby well but she still is not comfortable being a teen mother. She does not like taking the bus when she has the baby because of the looks people give her. She says she still loves Lee but he is slowly turning her love into disgust. Amy is also very hurt that he has not shown any care or responsibility for the baby. Though she does not plan to date boys for a while she still watches them. She does not like it that she can not go out without the baby, but is learning how to handle the situation.

Specific Goals and Plans

Amy is a typical immature fifteen year old at times, while at other times she is more mature and responsible than some adults. She plans to finish her high school education at Booth because Booth will assign her to her appropriate grade level next school year. She does not want to be dependent on a welfare check forever and plans to work. Amy realizes the limitations a baby poses when employed but she has applied for a summer job. She does not plan on getting married or having any more children. Both are unrealistic expectations but she has had no other alternates presented to her. She is going to use birth control to prevent any more unwanted pregnancies. I plan to offer her ideas about different life styles and continue our friendship.

As the interventions continued, the advocate found still further difficulties:

April 4

This week our schedules didn't work out but we did stay in contact. I talked to Amy on Wednesday and Friday. Saturday she wanted me to pick her up and take her to her aunt's house. I felt guilty, almost like I let her down, but I have to work and besides I'm not her free taxi service. I want to be there for her but not be taken advantage of.

By talking to her I found out she is supposed to go to court on April 9th to sign papers about who are the parents of the baby. She said that she is going to start to take the baby to school next week, and her social worker is interested in meeting me.

April 7

I talked to Amy today about her visit home last weekend. She said she took the baby down to show Lee and his family. She said Lee just looked at the baby real hard but he didn't pick him up. I asked her how she felt about going down there and letting Lee see the baby. She said it was all right but she didn't want to be there that long. I found out today that the court date was changed till April 14th instead of the 9th. I set up an appointment to meet her social worker next week and I'm going to be picking her up on Thursday from school. She told me that she really couldn't do too much with me anymore during the weekdays because her foster mom says she has too many things to do after school. She told me that she just doesn't get to do things like I do because she has a baby to take care of and I don't. I thought that was kind of cute.

April 9

I picked Amy up from school and took her home. She seemed to be complaining a lot about her foster mother. Amy said she won't let her go home and visit her family. She also told me the foster mother had a boyfriend who comes over during the day. I asked her if that bothered her and she said no, but she doesn't like to sit in the living room with them. She made some other complaints about how the foster mother never cleans or cooks. Sometimes I wonder how much of it is exaggerated. Amy tells me she doesn't get much sleep cause the baby keeps her up all night, and then her foster mother will wake her up early on days she can sleep in just to keep her (the foster mother) company. I tried to tell her that staying up all night is a part of taking care of the baby. And when I asked her if she really wanted to stay with her current foster mother, she said yes. I told her I got worried when she says everything is ok and it is better where she is than if she went to her other foster parent's home. I think that has a lot to do with being closer to her mom at the present house. I found a car seat that I can borrow until Amy buys one, or doesn't need one. I'll be keeping the seat in my car so if I pick her up with the baby I'll have it.

April 16

Yesterday I had a meeting with Amy's social worker, who filled me in on some of the rules their agency follows. We talked about Amy getting a new foster home and my relationship with her. It was an informative meeting for me and I'm glad I went.

Today I picked Amy and the baby up from school and we went shopping for a little while before she went to her group meeting. We talked about Lee a lot today. He didn't show up in court Tuesday and it really hurt to know he didn't care enough to show up. She said she still loves him but every time he does something like that she starts to dislike him more and more. Even though that court scene only happened two days ago she seemed really happy today. I was even teasing her about her looking at all the guys. She took back a new shirt and bought a pair of shoes to match the dress I gave her to wear for Easter. She wanted something nice to wear so I told her I had a dress if she wanted it. She liked it, and took back a shirt to buy the shoes. I explained to her why I haven't seen her as much as before and she understood. When I dropped her off she wanted to make sure we could get together next week. I would really like to have her come to my graduation, but we'll see. I'm really glad she is my little sister. I think we are getting along like real sisters would—she even irritates me sometimes just like my own sister does. I think that's actually good.

Many of the girls who most needed and wanted contact with a "big sister" were the most difficult to contact. Some had no telephone or fixed address. Some could be reached only at school, and, because of various problems—caring for younger siblings, transportation problems, ill health, or lack of motivation—they seldom attended school. Some were so burdened with home, work, and school demands that they were impossible to contact.

A peer advocate's journal shows a record of frustrated efforts to make contact:

FROM A JOURNAL: ANNE

January 29

After trying to meet with my two girls for two weeks one of them was finally in school. I met with my first girl, Anne, around 11:30. We talked for a few minutes and then I administered the questionnaire. We had to break for half an hour while she went to lunch, and then we picked up where we left off. After completing the questionnaire I explained to Anne what an MMPI was and asked her to complete it that evening and I would be by in the morning to pick it up. She then told me she would not be in school the next day but she would have it for me on Monday. We then discussed her likes and dislikes in entertainment, her school schedule and mine, and when and where would be the most convenient time for her to be picked up.

Before leaving I spoke to the women in the main office about Sara and was told she had not been in school that week but had good attendance.

February 4

I went to Booth to get Anne's MMPI and found that she was again not in school. I then talked to a woman in the office who told me she had never seen Anne but knew she was in trouble as she had heard teachers discussing her attendance problems. The woman then gave me Anne's telephone number. When I inquired about Sara she told me that Sara too had an attendance problem and that she had no phone number on file for the girl. On my way out I stopped by the attendance office and explained who I was and that I would like some information on Sara. They told me Sara had transferred to a different school over two months ago and gave me her current number.

This evening I called Sara in an attempt to set up a meeting. She told me she had never wanted to take part in the project, and despite my telling her of what we did, she still did not want to be part of it. I then told her to think it over and I would call her back in a few days.

The intervention included efforts to help the girls cope with the major life changes facing them and to transmit information. The girls seemed to appreciate these efforts but, often through no fault of their own, were unable to cooperate. Broken appointments were common. Two accounts, excerpted from the logs of two advocates, cast some light on the sources of this problem:

FROM A JOURNAL: MARY

March 5

After talking to Ms. Andrews it was decided that I should drop Anne and pick up a girl by the name of Mary. I tested the girl this afternoon and then gave her the MMPI to complete. We then talked for an hour about where she was living (Booth) and why (convenient, free medical care). She then told me she was going home that weekend so we could not go out, but agreed to have a late lunch with me before her ride picked her up.

March 6

I picked Mary up at 2:00 and asked her what she was in the mood for and she explained that she did not have any preference and knew of no restaurants in the area. I then decided to take her to the WSU area as I knew it was safe and we would have our choice of eating places. After walking into, and then out of 4 or 5 restaurants, we found one to Mary's liking. While we ate she talked about her mother, who is not married, completed 2 years at WSU before dropping out due to lack of interest, is unemployed and currently is living with her son in the Projects. Mary talked more about her aunt though than she did her mother. She did not mention specifics, just that the aunt took her more places than her mother did.

We then walked around the cultural center and Mary questioned me about college (was it hard, how long did it take).

We then headed back to Booth as her ride would be there shortly. As I was saying good-bye to Mary her social worker asked to see me. She told me that Mary was a good kid but needed a lot of support as she usually stayed at the Booth home and I guess rarely was home to visit her mother. She then told me if I ran into any problems to contact her and she would see if she could help.

March 11

On the way home from school I stopped in to see Mary and found out she was going to her boyfriend's mother's house for the weekend, but would like to go out with me again that coming Friday.

March 13

I picked Mary up for a ride today and we wound up stopping for ice cream. While we were riding around she talked about her boyfriend. They are committed to one another, and had planned on marrying in April, but have decided to move the date back. Right now he is elsewhere in the state, but Mary couldn't remember the correct name of the town. They do correspond by mail and his mother is taking Mary to see him tomorrow. She told me he is in a program where they take you away to a place and then train you for up to a year in a specific skill area.

I then got Mary to talk about what she wants to do. After the baby is born she wants to attend Booth for another year as she feels she is too weak in math. She then wants to attend a trade school to learn to be a secretary.

By then our time was over and I had to drop Mary off so she could pack. Before I left she agreed to have dinner with me the next Tuesday.

March 17

I picked Mary up at 5:00 and brought her over to my girlfriend's apartment where Mary and I had dinner with my fiancé. Over dinner we talked about school, and Mary told me she had made the honor roll. We all began discussing college and Mary told us she really had no desire to attend college. When we asked her why she said she had always wanted to be a secretary.

After dinner the three of us attended a movie of Mary's choice. She based her choice on the fact that the movie starred Michael J. Fox. After watching the movie we had to get her back as it was almost 10:00. On the way back to Booth, Mary started asking us about our getting married. We explained to her that we had set our date far enough into the future that we would be able to attain financial goals that would allow us to purchase a home and get ourselves established. Also, that we each had set career and school goals, and how we had arrived at these goals.

March 24

I went to get Mary today and found out she had left with some other girls from the school to go shopping.

March 27

I again stopped by to speak to Mary and caught her in the midst of packing for another weekend with her mother.

March 30

I went to Booth school today to get Mary and after being screened by 5 different people, I finally met with a social worker who told me Mary had not returned from the weekend with her mother.

FROM A JOURNAL: JANE

December 22

Jane and I had planned on going to a movie and restaurant to talk and see how she felt about the wedding but stood me up and didn't even call. This, I find, is one of the most frustrating parts of the entire intervention process. Jane has forgotten or not been able to make it home in time for our agreed upon time to enjoy some event together. I finally got her this evening at 8:30 pm. As before she just couldn't get back in time from the beauty parlor and taking a family picture with her mother. So as before all I can say is it's all right, we'll set up another time when she calls me later this week. But I get upset because I have to get a baby sitter for these times which Jane is aware of. Communication is one problem I see that may be an area we should help teenagers to see the importance of. I'll try again next week.

December 29

I tried to reach Jane because she has not returned my call as she said she would. All I get from her family is okay, I'll give her the message, but she doesn't return my calls. I leave my number each time because Jane has lost it three times already, but still no return call. I'll try again later this week!

January 11

I tried to reach Jane again and finally her mother-in-law told me she was out of town on her honeymoon and wouldn't return until January 18th, so I left a message for her to call when she returned.

January 20

I finally caught Jane at home and she was sorry of course for not letting me know she was going out of town. She let me know she had not returned to school until January 19th, although school started the second week of January. We talked about her getting behind in her class work, but she felt she could catch up and she didn't intend to stop going to school. I was glad to hear that because Jane has missed quite a few classes from school.

We made a date again, February 7th, at the Detroit Repertory Theater. I hope we make it this time. I do understand now, that teenagers usually don't have cars of their own so making appointments on time if at all isn't always up to them, but the person they are carpooling with. But this situation can be trying at times.

The intervention was a process of learning to communicate, to listen, to see life through another's eyes—both for the teens and for the big sisters. Each learned to know a different way of life. On the face of it, taking teenage girls to movies and plays does not sound like much more than providing entertainment. Intervention did not stop there, however. The experiences showed the girls a world and a way of life that could enrich or even replace what they had known. A dialogue began when the girls saw that someone would, perhaps for the first time in their lives, offer attention, genuine regard, and respect.

February 7

Well, what can I say, it doesn't look like Jane is going to make it to the theater this evening. I have called a few times this afternoon to confirm our arrangements about getting to the play by 8:15 pm and she hasn't been home and it is now 7:20 pm so I guess I will go to the theater alone. Jane finally calls at 7:45 pm to say she just couldn't get back before now and she got her time confused somehow because she though it was 6:45 pm. At this point I can't get to the far west side before 8:30 pm and the play starts at 8:30 pm. Jane said she will try to get a ride to the theater. So I arrived at the theater and left tickets for Jane, and also Karen (another peer advocate) and her girl, who are going to meet us at the play. At 8:30 pm the play began and still no Jane or Karen and her girl, so I went in. They all arrived at 9:00 pm. I was really relieved that they finally made it, and I could enjoy the production. We were not able to talk until the play was over because there was no intermission with the play. But afterward Jane really seemed to enjoy going to her first professional play. She asked questions about the theme of the play and whether or not the play was fiction or fact. The theater owner told us that the play was about a real American woman who returned to Germany and was arrested and tortured and she was able in real life to escape the prison and liked to write about the experience. Jane was so interested in the play that she asked me to make sure I invited her again to see another play when the next production started. I was happy to have opened up a whole new world of entertainment to Jane and Karen's girl. They both talked about it and how much they enjoyed seeing their first play.

December 9

I called Jane to see how her bridal shower plans were working out and how the wedding rehearsals were going. She was very excited and seemed pressed for time. She said she hadn't realized how much time, money, and energy all of the different events involved in getting to her wedding day would involve. Jane said trying to juggle school, spending time with her baby and fiancé and doing her job were extremely hard. Almost impossible, it seemed at times. But she was glad I called, because she hadn't realized how uptight she was getting from trying to get all the plans for the wedding to work out well. She said it was nice to have someone other than her family to talk about everything with because everybody in the family was busy trying to get ready for the bridal shower and wedding. I hadn't realized how sometimes just speaking on the phone sometimes helps her.

December 13

I have arrived at a bridal shower given for Jane by her aunt. Jane is very excited about all the pretty gifts she has received from her family and friends and all the love and support she has been given in pulling her coming wedding together. She is especially glad that I have come because we haven't been friends that long and she appreciates my taking the time to share and talk about how she feels about getting married. We discussed the difficulties she was having with her parents because the baby's father was not of their religion. She finally had to move in to her fiancé's home with his mother and brothers and sisters. Following her move into her fiancé's home the two of them decided to get married earlier than anticipated because they were now living together.

We are now having fun doing all the silly games you play at a bridal shower, like seeing how many cotton balls you can scoop out of a bowl with a spoon and put them in another bowl while you're in blind folds. I really felt Jane and I are becoming closer friends because I could share an event that was important to her and a major turning point in her life.

December 20

I attended Jane's wedding and what a beautiful event. Her dress was lovely, and she looked like a queen. You could see how happy and relieved she was that the special day had arrived. I was able to meet her mother and brothers and sister. Everybody seemed to have worked out the differences of opinions now that the wedding was about to be completed. I didn't get a chance to talk to Jane too long because she was so excited and nervous; but she did say she was happy I could share this important day with her.

Later that evening I arrived at the wedding reception party and had a lot of fun dancing and eating. I was able to talk for a short time with Jane's husband, who seems to really love her and his son. From this conversation it seems he wants Jane to finish high school and go to college if she really wants to.

Jane continued to keep up in school, care for her baby, work part time, attend to household duties, and remain active with church activities. Her peer advocate found it increasingly difficult to meet with Jane, since there was virtually no spare time in Jane's busy schedule. They maintained contact by phone through most of the spring, and Jane confided that these frequent calls helped her cope with the many demands she faced. At last it was time to graduate.

June 6

Today I met Jane and her family at the graduation at Booth. It was a beautiful ceremony and all the girls and their babies were dressed up and excited. It was the first time I had seen Jane since March, and she was truly radiant. I was so proud of her for completing school while bearing so many responsibilities at home. I had a chance to talk with her during the reception afterwards, and she told me how much our relationship had meant to her and that she hoped I would continue to call her occasionally. I gave her and the baby a big hug, telling her again and again how proud everyone was of her. On the way home I felt strangely sad and let down. The year has been rewarding, and despite the frustration I've experienced in trying to get together with Jane, I know I will miss her.

FROM A JOURNAL: SANDY

November 19

I went to Sandy's house today to administer the MMPI. I explained the test to her and reminded her that I would watch her son, Dylan, while she took the test. Sandy is 16 years old and Dylan is just 5 months. He is small for his age, but since he was a month premature it isn't too surprising that he is still catching up. He was very responsive to me, smiling and looking at my face. He tried to creep to reach me and didn't seem shy at all despite my being a stranger to him. Sandy was surprised that he was being so good because he has a cold and had been very cranky. She seems proud of him and likes to hear people say complimentary things about him.

Later on Sandy's mom came home from work and said she had been wanting to meet me. She asked about the peer advocate class I take at Wayne and expressed concern about the project and Sandy's part in it. She thought I would befriend Sandy only as long as my grade depended on it, then I would drop Sandy and that would be the end of it. I explained to her that I hope to build a friendship with Sandy, as well as help her adjust to her new responsibilities. Sandy's mother appreciated hearing that I hope to continue a friendship with Sandy even after the project ends, and I think she realized that the project really is intended to help the girls, not just treat them as cases in files. I can understand her concern. I know what it is like to have friends to count on and then sometimes be let down when they move away or find new activities.

December 31

I called Sandy, and asked if she was going to be home that afternoon and she said she was. I told her I would like to stop by to see her.

When I came in, Dylan (her baby) was in the crib surrounded with tons of toys, crying his head off. Sandy said he's constipated and the medicine the doctor gave him is not taking its effect.

Also, I notice that in the middle of the room was a kerosene heater. The window sills were covered with rolled up towels and so was the door, so drafts wouldn't get in. I told Sandy that kerosene gives off fumes and the fumes can be hazardous. She said she knows that and they don't use it often unless it gets really cold. Sandy also mentioned the house is old and drafty, and the owner controls the heat stingily.

I brought Sandy her Christmas present. It was a vest with purple stripes against an off white background. She really liked it (I think) and she put it on—in case the size wasn't the right one.

She told me she has been going to the doctor because Dylan can't seem to get rid of his cold, is not acting well, and losing quite a bit of weight. The doctor gave her some cold medicine and a food supplement.

She showed me her Christmas gifts and how surprised she was to receive so many gifts. She was really grateful because most of the gifts were for her personal use—clothes, under clothes, socks, and Avon perfume. She thought her relatives and friends would just give her stuff for the baby. But she got some gifts and so did the baby.

I encouraged Sandy to try to get a safer heater, or at least ventilate the room occasionally. I also reminded her that the school could provide information about who to contact to get help for heating costs. I offered to drive her to the next doctor's appointment for Dylan so she wouldn't have to take the bus.

FROM A JOURNAL: DONNA

March 22

I called Donna to ask her if she wanted to go out to Belle Isle for a little stroll. I really wanted to talk to her and get to know her a little bit, and most of all get her to talk to me. Our first meeting was a disaster, she wouldn't initiate any level of conversation—it was a question and answer episode.

Donna's house was in a rugged neighborhood—there were several abandoned buildings, ransacked and weren't boarded. She was all set to go and Danny (her son) was in the stroller. Her mom came out of the bedroom, I said "Hello" and she just walked past me with a stone face. Then she and Donna went to the kitchen and started yelling. Donna couldn't get in a word. I overheard her mom describing what I'm doing with her as "charity." Donna came out of the kitchen trying not to cry, and told me she couldn't go. No reason. And she made it clear that I can't come over to her house or call her. If I want to get in touch with her I have to go to Booth.

March 25

I went to Booth when school was letting out. When Donna saw me, she was a little bit surprised. She said hi and I told her I'd drop her home. Before we left Booth we sat in the car and talked. I asked Donna if I could stop by and talk to her mom and explain to her who I am, what I'm doing, and most of all apologize about Sunday's fiasco. Donna just said, "You didn't do anything, she's always like that, changing her mind or not remembering." I told Donna that I like her and would like to take her out sometime. She seemed to like the idea. Also, I told her whenever we go out I'll call her a few days in advance and to remind her mother of our date to avoid further mix-up.

From the journal entries it is evident that the intervention process was not without difficulties. Initially, some of the teens refused to cooperate with the interview and the MMPI by failing to attend school on the appointed day. Scheduling activities with the girls was sometimes difficult due to everyone's busy schedules. Particularly problematic was the fact that the teens chosen as those most in need of intervention were the ones who typically did not attend school. It was often extremely difficult to contact them, and sometimes they had returned to their former schools without notifying anyone at the Booth School that they were leaving. Several advocates asked to be removed from the project due to many such frustrations.

The safety of the peer advocates was always a concern and one that was addressed regularly. When possible, advocates were advised to pick their little sisters up from the Booth School during daylight hours and take them home in the early evening. Similarly, weekend outings during the daytime were encouraged. Because many of the teenage mothers lived in less desirable neighborhoods, it was sometimes necessary for advocates to work in pairs, taking their girls out together.

One advocate faced a very difficult situation one night when her little sister called her to say that she had just ingested an overdose of medication. Concerned about the girl, the advocate pressed for her location, called the police, and went with her mother to the scene. After waiting for the police to no avail, they tried to convince the teen (who was with her boyfriend) to go with them to the hospital. This resulted in the girl becoming rather combative, at which point the advocate's mother insisted that they return home.

The incident raised concern among the project staff for the advocates' welfare and their responsibility in such incidents. Again, the need for imparting to the teen mothers an awareness of social resources was underscored. When the same adolescent called her advocate several months later feeling suicidal, the advocate encouraged her to call the suicide hotline, which she did.

At the close of the school year most peer advocates indicated that they wished to maintain contact with their little sisters. Possibly this in itself was a stage of intervention, because it expressed to the teens as nothing else could that they were respected as people whose feelings deserved consideration. For some teens, whose lives had been filled with loneliness, rejection, and instability, the realization that they were liked might have been a milestone in their lives.

Many of the problems connected with the teen pregnancy and parenthood, including the incidence of teen pregnancy itself, have been shown to be related to low self-esteem in teen girls. This crucial factor is one that cannot be addressed by educational programs alone. It may also have a role in keeping youngsters from seeking help from school counselors and walk-in clinics. It is hoped that intensive, individual social support intervention may help increase girls' self-esteem. If we are able to communicate to teen girls that they are valued, worthwhile human beings, then educational and vocational interventions may have a better chance of being effective.

Chapter 6

Preventing Teen Pregnancy

From a journal:

> Today while we were at the park, Carol confided that this was not her first pregnancy. When she was 14 she got pregnant by a boy she had only gone out with once. She was too scared to tell her mother about it so she threw herself down a flight of stairs hoping to have a miscarriage. She was successful.
>
> Now that she has Cassandra (from her second pregnancy) she still has lots of problems. She told me it drives her crazy when the baby cries all the time. She can't go anywhere because she has to take Cassandra with her and that's just too much trouble. She seems very depressed to me and I'm worried about her. Maybe what bothers me the most is that Carol and her new boyfriend are sexually active, but Carol doesn't use birth control. We've talked about it, but Carol always seems to try to change the subject. I think her boyfriend is against the idea of her using birth control. She told me once that it bugs him that the baby isn't his. He wants her to have *his* baby.

Despite the negative consequences of teenage pregnancy and the difficulties young mothers face in rearing a child, the incidence of sexual activity and pregnancy in adolescents has continued to rise. Chapter 1 discussed the psychological and psychosocial variables associated with teen-age pregnancy as well as many of the reasons young girls give for not using contraception. While not intended to be redundant, this chapter will begin with a brief overview of the basic models of contraceptive risk-taking be-haviors and then discuss prevention strategies and specific interventions designed to enhance contraceptive awareness and use among adolescents.

MODELS OF CONTRACEPTIVE RISK-TAKING BEHAVIOR

Contraceptive Ignorance

Several models explaining contraceptive risk-taking behavior have been described in the literature (Gerrard, McCann, & Fortini, 1983; Hogan, Astone, & Kitagawa, 1985; Hogan & Kitagawa, 1985). The contraceptive ignorance model suggests that adolescents who engage in unprotected sex-ual intercourse lack adequate information regarding contraception and reproduction. It follows from this perspective that improved sex education courses, which offer information regarding human sexuality, birth control, and reproduction, would be needed. However, recent studies dispute this model or at least indicate that it is an incomplete solution (Gerrard et al., 1983; Lindemann & Scott, 1981). One study of pregnant teens in New Orleans (Landry, Bertrand, Cherry, & Rice, 1986) found that although more than 86% reported knowing about contraceptives, and almost 75% stated that they knew where to get them, only 16% reported using them at the time they got pregnant. In this study those who used contraceptives did know about a greater number of methods, their correct usage, and more about availability, but the childbearers still knew a mean number of four methods. This suggests a disparity between knowledge and its imple-mentation into practice.

Personality Variables

A second model focuses on aspects of personality, hypothesizing that al-though adolescents have adequate knowledge regarding birth control meth-ods, certain characteristics prevent them from successfully utilizing the knowledge. Several personality variables have been found to relate to the effective use of contraceptives. For example, those with guilt regarding sexuality tend to be poor contraceptors (Gerrard, 1987). Such guilt appears to lead certain women to feel uncomfortable about their decision to engage in sexual relations, and, while this guilt is thought to be strong enough to limit their planning and preparing for sexual relations, it does not stop them from engaging in intercourse. Poor planning ability (Mindick, Os-kamp, & Berger, 1977) may also predispose adolescents to sexual risk-taking behavior. Individuals who are good contraceptors show significantly longer future time extension (i.e., they think about and plan for the future), while poor contraceptors tend to view future events more negatively. In addition, holding an external locus of control may predispose adolescents to believe that fate and chance, rather than their own behaviors, will influence the outcome of their sexual activities (Bolton, 1980).

Cognitive Model

According to the cognitive model, contraceptive behavior is mediated by cognitive variables, including thoughts, attitudes, and beliefs regarding contraception and pregnancy. From this perspective, positive attitudes toward parenthood and negative attitudes toward contraception would predispose individuals to contraceptive risk-taking behavior. Gerrard et al. (1983) substantiated these hypotheses in a study of college females. They also found that ineffective contraceptors who did not become pregnant attributed it to a low probability of conception. In the study, good and poor contraceptors showed no differences regarding knowledge of birth control methods.

Further support for this model is suggested by adolescents' level of cognitive development (Jorgenson, 1981). While they may be moving toward the abstraction involved in formal operations, adolescents tend to hold certain characteristic modes of thinking. Their thinking is egocentric (Elkind, 1967), and a strong preoccupation with themselves leads to the assumption of the imaginary audience and personal fable (see chapter 1). There is evidence that these two types of thinking play a part in decisions not to use birth control. Cvetkovitch, Grote, Bjorseth, and Sarkissian (1975) suggest that adolescents believe that planning for sexual relations by using contraceptives will disclose their sexuality to scrutiny by themselves and the imaginary audience. Their insecurities regarding their sexuality do not allow them to withstand this scrutiny or to admit an acceptance of their sexual behavior. The personal fable allows them to hold erroneous beliefs—for example, that they are immune to pregnancy, that they are sterile, or that no particular coital episode will lead to pregnancy.

It has been suggested that adolescents have not reached the level of cognitive development to be able to develop genuine intimacy, to understand the complexities of mature sexual relationships, or to properly practice birth control (Pestrak & Martin, 1985). This raises important questions regarding the focus of sex education programs. It implies that learning about birth control methods would not be sufficient to allow adolescents to act properly on such knowledge (Jorgenson, 1981).

While there is evidence for cognitions holding an important role in decisions regarding sexual activity and contraceptive use, the model appears to be an incomplete solution due to findings of inconsistencies between cognitions, or attitudes, and actual behavior. Although many adolescents hold attitudes toward pregnancy and birth control that are consistent with their behavior, there is a large minority for whom the behavior and attitudes are clearly at variance (Zabin, Hirsch, Smith, & Hardy, 1984). Zabin et al. found that of sexually experienced adolescents 83% reported a best age for first intercourse as older than the age at which they first engaged in it, 43% reported an age older than their current stated age, and 39% of females and 32% of males view premarital sex as wrong. In addition, 25% of those who reported that they would have sex only if they were using birth control also reported that they did not use it during their last intercourse. These findings suggest a role for motivational factors that may supercede cognitive beliefs.

Social and Environmental Factors

A fourth model suggests that social and environmental factors contribute to teen pregnancy and decreased contraceptive use. Black teens who live in metropolitan areas of the United States tend to begin sexual intercourse earlier and to have higher rates of premarital pregnancy (Hogan & Kitagawa, 1985). A survey of sexually active black females in Chicago (Hogan, Astone, & Kitagawa, 1985) found that coming from a low socioeconomic background, living in a ghetto, growing up in female-headed families with a large number of children, and having one or more sisters who were teen mothers are risk factors for early sexual behavior without adequate contraception and premarital pregnancy. It is suggested that in such an environment career aspirations are low and parents are unable to adequately monitor initial dating among their children, which contributes to the higher degree of risk. Hogan and Kitagawa (1985) found that black teenagers from this type of high-risk environment are 8.3 times more likely to become pregnant than are girls from lower-risk environments.

Another indication that sociocultural factors play an important role in contraceptive practices is obtained from findings that the United States is among the countries having the highest rate of adolescent childbearing (Westhoff, Calot, & Foster, 1983). Racial factors do not fully account for these findings; although the fertility rate for blacks is high in the United States, the fertility rate for whites here is still higher than the fertility rate in all but four countries studied. Speculations about the reasons for this, such as a reliance on abortion in other countries or financial incentives such as support from the Aid to Families with Dependent Children program in the United States, do not appear to explain the findings adequately. Other countries, such as Sweden, offer better support for single-parent families but show lower rates of premarital pregnancy. Brown (1983), in describing attitudes toward sex and sex education in Sweden, implies that an acknowledgment of adolescents' rights to make responsible decisions about sexuality, and an approach that helps adolescents clarify their values, may contribute to increased contraceptive use.

REASONS FOR ADOLESCENT PREGNANCY

Each model described above, except perhaps the contraceptive ignorance model, raises questions regarding the motivation for pregnancy by those who become pregnant. One study of pregnant adolescents found, by their own self-report, that two thirds had wanted to become pregnant and have a child. The remaining individuals reported that they did not want a child but became pregnant due to unforeseen circumstances (Lindemann & Scott, 1981). Others (Zelnik & Kantner, 1978) found that 30% to 40% had planned their pregnancies, suggesting that a significant number of pregnant teens acted purposefully to have a child. Lindemann and Scott (1981) found differences in contraceptive behavior between the two groups. For example, those who did not want to become pregnant were more likely to have discussed sex and birth control with teachers, sisters, or girlfriends.

Reasons for wanting a child during adolescence fall under both psychological and sociocultural factors. Babies may represent hope, not just for the individuals but also for society (Rickel, 1986). A baby may fill a psychological need for a love object, affection, or attachment (Bolton, 1980; Lindemann & Scott, 1981). For some teens getting pregnant may be an assertion of dependency or of a girl's own need to be mothered and a way of gaining attention (Hatcher, 1976). Alternately, an adolescent may feel that having a baby will help her assert autonomy from or rebel against parents, especially if parent-adolescent relations are strained or filled with conflict (Bolton, 1980; Joffe, 1986).

For lower-class women, becoming a mother may be a means to become socialized, achieve adult status, and reach maturity. Girls of lower socioeconomic status are often thought to hold beliefs that minimize the social consequences of or even provide positive sanctions for becoming a mother. They are also less likely to envision alternatives to the traditional motherhood role and tend to have few prospects for other forms of achievement. Their sense of hopelessness or even boredom may be dissipated by the prospect of becoming a mother (Hogan & Kitagawa, 1985; Lindemann & Scott, 1981).

Findings such as these indicate the complexity of the problem of teenage pregnancy and the likelihood of a multidimensional causal model. There have been a variety of programs and research projects regarding prevention and intervention. Unmarried adolescent mothers have few economic, social, or emotional resources and are therefore considered at risk for problems with childrearing and for repeat pregnancies. The likelihood of an adolescent mother having a second child within a brief period is quite high. Blacks who are younger at their first childbirth are more likely to have their next child quickly. At all ages Hispanics who have a first child are more likely than blacks or whites to have a second child quickly. Other variables that relate to repeat pregnancies in adolescence include having a mother who dropped out of high school, wanting the first child at the time of conception, and being married at the time of the first birth (Mott, 1986).

These findings are important in light of the social and economic consequences of adolescent childrearing. They have resulted in the administration of many programs that have attempted to help teen mothers cope better with their children by enhancing their parenting skills (Rickel, 1986), such as the Detroit Teen Parent Project, described earlier. Apparently important aspects of this program include the individualized attention the young mothers are receiving by remaining in a school program, in addition to training in child development issues and childrearing practices. Other programs have attempted to specifically refocus the lives of these teens into more productive channels (Polit & Kahn, 1985). It is also suggested that adolescent fathers are in need of counseling, job training, and social support to assist in breaking this cycle (Stark, 1986).

Project Redirection (Polit & Kahn, 1985) is a program with comprehensive services to move the lives of disadvantaged young mothers onto a path of economic self-sufficiency. It offers employment training, education regarding the development of relationships with service providers, peer group sessions, and relationships with community women. Girls in the program showed some decline in repeat pregnancies; increases in contraceptive use, school attendance, and graduation; and an increased likelihood to hold a job. These findings were more positive for those who were initially the most disadvantaged. There is some indication, however, that these positive gains dissipate once the program terminates, suggesting the need for continuance of longer programs.

A true primary prevention model, however, would work to start earlier, by targeting those teens considered at high risk for becoming premaritally pregnant. The task of reducing the pregnancy rate of adolescents requires intervention at two stages. The first involves decreasing the number of sexual relations and may partially be accomplished by delaying the onset of sexual activities until older ages (Hogan & Kitagawa, 1985). The second is to increase the use or effectiveness of contraceptives when sexual relations do occur (Jorgenson, 1981). Although some adolescent pregnancies may result from individual factors, a large proportion are the result of a cultural code in which adolescent motherhood is considered normative. In such instances to focus on the problem as one that resides wholly at the individual level would seriously undercut effective preventive efforts (Sameroff, Seifer, Zax, & Barocas, 1987). It appears, therefore, that prevention efforts must be conducted at both individual and environmental levels.

SEX EDUCATION

One of the primary formats used in the attempt to deal with the issues of teenage sexuality and contraception has been through sex education courses in the schools. The central goal of these programs has been to decrease the teenage pregnancy rate, but subsumed under this have been attempts to encourage more responsible and competent decision-making; provide accurate information regarding sexually transmitted diseases, reproduction, sexuality, and contraception; facilitate rewarding sexual expression; and reduce fears and anxieties about personal sexual development and feelings (Kirby, Alter, & Scales, 1979). One problem with these programs is that the quality and focus of sex education courses around the country vary considerably, with no formal definition of what the courses should consist of or what the effective ingredients might be.

Suggestions for improving sex education programs may be obtained by examining the approach used in Sweden, where there has been a consistent decrease in teen pregnancy since a peak in 1974. Alternately, there has been a 12% increase in the teen pregnancy rate in the United States between 1974 and 1983 (Brown, 1983). Sex education has been compulsory in Sweden since 1956, and a nationwide revised curriculum was implemented in 1977 that emphasized teaching sexuality in the context of personal relationships and their psychological, ethical, and social dimensions. In the new curriculum, much emphasis was placed on values in order to help adolescents develop their own value systems and goals for personal relationships. While certain fundamental values (e.g., rejection of sexual violence) are stressed, more controversial topics (e.g., abortion, premarital sex) are taught from a value-free perspective; that is, the issues and alternatives are explicitly discussed, but no specific position is taken by the teachers. The curriculum takes a pragmatic approach, with an acceptance that the majority of adolescents are sexually active, and a focus on the taking of responsibility. In elementary grades the topic of contraception is brought up, but actual techniques are discussed in later grades in an attempt to place the use of contraceptives into a natural context.

In a positive comparison of programs in the United States and Sweden, a study of U.S. sex education programs (Kirby et al., 1979) indicated that the most successful ones combined education regarding reproduction with values and attitudes regarding dating, relationships, and life goals. Other aspects of effective programs included peer counseling and parental involvement.

Studies of sex education courses (Dawson, 1986; Marsiglio & Mott, 1986; Zelnik & Kim, 1982) have consistently found no relationship between having taken a sex education course and decisions regarding initiation of sexual activity. While this does serve to negate conservative notions that learning or talking about sex will lead adolescents to have sex, it also raises questions about the usefulness of these courses in preventing intercourse. More promising is that there is an increased likelihood for those who have taken sex education courses to use birth control during their first sexual experience (Dawson, 1986; Zelnik & Kim, 1982) and overall (Marsiglio & Mott, 1986). While Zelnik and Kim found that those who took sex education courses were less likely to become pregnant, the two 1986 studies found no significant relationship between taking a course and the likelihood of becoming premaritally pregnant.

Other suggestions for improving sex education courses involve improving the quality and training of sex education instructors (Jorgenson, 1981), using peer tutors to model and reinforce knowledge, developing a standardized program based on further empirical investigations, and gearing programs more specifically to the level of adolescents' cognitive development. Jorgenson (1981) points out that there is a potential mismatch between the content or teaching methods used in these courses and the ability of adolescents to understand, integrate, or internalize the information. He suggests direct confrontation of the personal fables described above and more personalized discussion taking the adolescents' level of egocentrism into account. In line with this, Steinlauf (1979) suggests teaching more effective means-end problem-solving, with a focus on the potential for a variety of possible solutions. Indicating that solving problems associated with sexual behavior and birth control is no different from solving other daily problems is thought to offer teens a sense of control and improve reasoning, judgment, and subsequently contraceptive effectiveness.

Other areas to alter involve the content of material and information that is provided to students, regardless of whether this is done through sex education courses or at family planning clinics. One issue to take into account is that adolescents, especially younger ones, are more likely to engage in sexual activity on an irregular basis. Taking the pill on a daily basis may therefore seem irrelevant and missing a day might seem like no big deal. Therefore, a focus on knowledge and on becoming comfortable using alternative methods may be more useful with this age group (Freeman, Rickels, Mudd, & Huggins, 1982).

Another area of concern for individuals engaging in sexual relations is that of contracting sexually transmitted diseases. The recent and growing spread of acquired immunodeficiency syndrome (AIDS) makes this an even more crucial issue. One means of protection against transmission of the AIDS virus, besides abstinence, that is being stressed is the use of condoms.

Educators may be able to motivate some adolescents who are ambivalent about using condoms by pointing out this serious threat to their health.

FAMILY PLANNING CLINICS

Another method of attempting to help adolescents obtain contraceptives has been to develop family planning clinics specifically geared toward them. One such clinic was a 3-year experimental program that was hospital based in the Columbia-Presbyterian Medical Center in New York City (Jones, Namerow, & Philliber, 1982). The Adolescent Reproductive Health Care Program was designed to meet the needs of an inner-city, low-income population and incorporated a variety of family planning, obstetric-gyne-cological, and postpartum services as well as the additional Young Adult Clinic set up as part of this study. Specific steps were taken to attempt to remove barriers that might have decreased adolescent attendance. These steps included holding late afternoon and evening hours, with walk-in scheduling as opposed to prearranged appointments; simple admissions procedures; subsidized services based on ability to pay; guaranteeing confidentiality without requiring parental consent; anonymity, since the clinic was part of a large medical complex; location in a central and accessible area; and hiring staff and volunteers who matched the ethnic and cultural backgrounds of the clientele and who were specifically trained to work with adolescents. Counselors were recruited from the surrounding communities to assist in education programs, and the staff did much outreach work as well as individual counseling and therefore became familiar with the patients. Their outreach work included assisting in sex education classes in nearby junior high schools and with church and community groups that discussed family planning. There was a large increase in the use of these services throughout the time of the program, indicating that the program was attracting adolescents and that a hospital is a feasible place for such a program. However, Jones et al.'s evaluation methods did not allow them to distinguish which aspects of the program were most helpful or the actual effect on pregnancy rates. Since the pregnancy rate in surrounding communities remained quite high, it appears that further efforts should be made toward attracting adolescents at even younger ages and that more follow-up regarding use of contraceptives be done.

Some researchers have examined the usefulness of community family planning clinics that are not specifically geared toward serving adolescents. It was found (Kisker, 1984) that Planned Parenthood clinics are more effective than other types of facilities, while with respect to increasing birth control use community action programs and neighborhood health centers ranked highest in terms of levels of patient satisfaction and patient reten-tion. Mid-sized clinics and nonmetropolitan clinics were also found to be more effective. Factors that were considered helpful with adolescents involved several of those incorporated into the previously described program in New York City. These included holding community education programs for adolescents, enlisting the support of local churches and youth groups, opening the clinic during evenings and weekends, scheduling walk-in hours, locating clinics in nearby neighborhoods, and increasing the time spent with each patient to decrease their resistance and discuss their concerns regarding contraception and sexuality.

SCHOOL-BASED FAMILY PLANNING CLINICS

Quite a few programs have combined school and sex education courses with family planning clinic programs and have shown promise for increasing the use of contraceptives and decreasing pregnancy rates. These services were initiated in response to findings that the rate of birth control use increases with easy access to birth control services (Hogan et al., 1985). In addition, from the clinic staff's perspective, school-based clinics provide easy access to students for performing adequate follow-up counseling (Ralph & Edgington, 1983).

The first of these school-based or school-related programs was developed in St. Paul-Minneapolis, in 1973 (Dryfoos, 1985; Edwards, Steinman, Arnold, & Hakanson, 1980). It began as part of the St. Paul Maternal and Infant Care (MIC) Project, which soon added prenatal and postpartum care, along with other reproductive health services in an inner-city junior-senior high school. Soon after it began, the project started to offer a wider range of health services to broaden its appeal and reduce the stigma for those attending the clinic. New services included physical examinations, immunizations, and weight control programs. The program gradually expanded its size and range of programs. It is now located in four high schools in St. Paul, serves three quarters of all students, and includes services such as dental care and a day care center. Simple laboratory and pregnancy tests are done onsite. Although sex education, examinations, and follow-up are provided at the school clinic, students are referred to an afterschool clinic at a nearby medical center to obtain contraceptives. To provide continuity of care and familiarity, however, the afterschool clinic is also staffed by those who work at the school clinics. The staff includes a nurse practitioner, social worker, and technician as well as a part-time nutritionist, pediatric nurse, pediatrician, and obstetrician-gynecologist. The program reports a significant decline in births and high contraceptive continuation rates among participating students. Between 1973 and 1976 there was a 56% decline in fertility, from 79 to 35 births per 1,000 students at the junior-senior high school that served as a pilot school. There was a decrease from 60 pregnancies per 1,000 students in 1976 to 46 per 1,000 in 1979 and 26 per 1,000 in 1983 for the more recent high school programs. In addition, since the program began, there have been fewer repeat pregnancies and pregnant teens are more likely to remain in school.

There are a growing number of comprehensive health service clinics, including family planning services, in or near public high schools and junior high schools. Most other programs have followed the pattern of the Minneapolis program, although there is considerable variation among them. Dryfoos (1985) summarized the services of 14 of these programs, which typically have been located in low-income urban neighborhoods. Most serve only their students, although some are able to assist recent graduates or school dropouts. Caseloads include from one quarter to three quarters of all students at the schools, with equal numbers of males and females attending.

As comprehensive health care clinics, these programs offer a wide range of services, including physical examinations; treatment for minor acute illnesses, accidents, and injuries; laboratory tests; screening for sexually transmitted diseases; nutrition information; and referrals to social service agencies. Most also have programs for weight loss, treatment of drug and alcohol abuse, dental services, immunization, individual and family counseling, and a variety of other services.

Family planning services are also rather complete. Regardless of their reason for attending the clinic, most new patients are asked about sexual activity and encouraged to make use of family planning services and to use contraceptives if they are sexually active. The clinics offer individual counseling about sexuality, gynecological examinations, and follow-up exams. Some offer contraceptive prescriptions, and some refer to off-site birth control clinics. A few dispense contraceptives onsite and follow up users at home by telephone. Ideally, the same nurse practitioner who makes a referral to an outside agency will also work in that agency to provide continuity. Many programs offer sex education to groups at the clinic, do pregnancy testing, and offer prenatal care. In some schools, classroom sex education or health education is provided through the program by the same nurse practitioner who works at the clinic. This helps link health education and clinic services.

Follow-up is easy, since the staff has access to students while they are in school. Staff may call students to the clinic while maintaining confidentiality, since they could be called to the health clinic for any number of reasons. Confidentiality is stressed, but often parental consent is required. Many schools try to gain blanket consent from parents for use of the clinic, without having them specify or know what services their adolescents are using.

Most such programs were started by an individual outside the school system (i.e., someone affiliated with a local public health agency or a voluntary health organization, physicians based at local teaching hospitals or community health centers), but the cooperation of principals and teachers is vital. Community support is also important. Most programs are funded by private foundations; monetary and in-kind donations are also obtained from schools, health care providers, or other groups. Public funds are sought from state departments of maternal and child health, social services, and education, among others, to keep the programs running. In some programs, Medicaid reimbursement can be obtained for health services.

Empirical evaluation of these programs has been limited, although there is some evidence that they help improve students' general health, lower birthrates, raise levels of contraceptive use, and improve school attendance. Still, these findings are tentative since there have been few reliable studies, and there is a strong need for better evaluation and monitoring of the programs.

Researchers at the Johns Hopkins School of Medicine's Department of Pediatrics and Department of Gynecology and Obstetrics (Zabin, Hardy, Streett, & King, 1984; Zabin, Hirsch, Smith, Streett, & Hardy, 1986a, 1986b) developed and administered a school-based program among inner-city, low-socioeconomic-status, black adolescents. This program was specifically designed to include an evaluation component, which is an essential difference between this and many other programs. The program served one junior high school and one senior high school in the Baltimore, Maryland, school system. In addition, one junior high school and one senior high school served as controls. The program provided education in sexuality and contraceptives, individual and group counseling, and medical and contraceptive services for a period of almost 3 school years. The focus of the program was on the development of personal responsibility, goal-setting, and communication with parents about sexuality and contraceptive use. Although the program provided education regarding sexuality, sex education courses normally taught in the respective schools remained as usual.

An evaluative component that examined changes in knowledge, attitudes, and behavior of the students was built into the program. Data collection was accomplished through self-administered questionnaires that were completed once before the program began and again in the spring term of each of the following 3 years. There were several methodological problems related to the use of school students, including dropout due to school transfers; initial data being collected in the fall, and later data in the spring term when attendance is lower; school differences; and differences due to the ages, grades, and length of time students were exposed to the program.

Several changes resulted from the program that are indicative of its usefulness. There was a significant, although not dramatic, increase in knowledge about contraceptives and the risks of pregnancy in the program schools but not the nonprogram schools. The findings regarding changes in attitudes, such as acceptance of teenage pregnancy and the best age to have children, were slight and inconsistent, suggesting that attitudes are harder to change than knowledge. There were also positive changes in contraceptive behavior in these schools, which at baseline had high levels of sexual activity. First, attendance at the clinic increased rapidly throughout the program, and by the end of the second year 41% of sexually active junior high school females and 58% of sexually active high school females had made use of it. Attendance at the clinic was related to an overall decrease in unprotected sexual activity. More specifically, there was some delay in initiation of first intercourse, a higher percentage of visits to the clinic before first intercourse, increased usage of the pill and other methods that require advance preparation, and low levels of no contraceptive use at last intercourse in those who attended the clinic. Of students who had attended the program for 2 or more years, less than 20% reported engaging in intercourse without contraceptives as opposed to 44 to 49% of students in the nonprogram school. Overall, there were more dramatic changes in the younger students, who may have had less sexual exposure prior to utilizing the program. This emphasizes the need for intervention at even younger ages.

There were decreases in pregnancy rates in the program schools in grades 9 through 12. Results indicated that after 16 months of exposure there was a 13% increase in pregnancy rates in program schools compared to a 50% increase in nonprogram schools, after 20 months there was a 22.5% decrease compared to a 39.5% increase, and after 28 months there was a 30.1% decrease compared to a 57% increase, respectively, in the program and nonprogram schools. In making these analyses, there are the factors of increased likelihood to engage in sexual activity as the students get older, while also being exposed to the program for longer periods of time. Although lower sexual activity in the earlier grades limited the analyses, there appeared to be small reductions in pregnancy rates for girls aged 15 and younger.

Overall, this program reports success in increasing the use of contraception, delaying the onset of sexual intercourse, and decreasing pregnancy rates. A longer evaluation and exposure period would offer more definitive findings. Still the strong findings with younger students, as well as improvements related to length of exposure to the program, suggest the importance of even earlier intervention (Zabin et al., 1986a). This is stressed further by the finding that, in general, younger adolescents are more likely to fail to use contraceptives (Mindick et al., 1977).

A summary of the positive aspects of this type of school-based health clinic approach includes (1) easy accessibility, since health services are provided in or near schools where adolescents are located; (2) consistent attention from staff; (3) combining of health education in classes with actual medical treatment; (4) high-quality, free services; (5) with family planning and health services combined, students can obtain contraception without being labeled as sexually active; (6) an array of health services; and (7) possible improvement in general health and therefore attendance (Dryfoos, 1985; Zabin et al., 1986a). There have been a number of problems or limitations of the program as well: (1) bureaucratic, staffing, and organizational problems; (2) funding uncertainties; (3) touchiness regarding counseling about abortion; and (4) many programs are only in operation during school hours. Overall, however, the clinics appear to be quite popular with students. Those who are involved with them hope that they may eventually be integrated into the school system itself, in a way similar to guidance offices (Dryfoos, 1985).

ADDITIONAL AREAS OF CONCERN AND PREVENTIVE STRATEGIES

The complexity of factors influencing adolescent sexuality and contraceptive use necessitates consideration of adolescent pregnancies within a broad context, including the adolescent's level of cognitive and emotional development, relationships with family and peers, and understanding of sexuality and gender-linked norms for sexual behavior within particular sociocultural contexts. Preventive efforts would therefore address adolescents' rapid rise in sexual activity and help them delay involvements until they are ready to express their feelings in responsible and self-enhancing ways, attempt to challenge cultural myths about gender and sexuality, and help them balance responsibilities toward themselves and their partners. For minority teens, social changes that provide more meaningful educational experiences and more inviting work opportunities as impetus to defer parenthood are needed (Maracek, 1987).

Currently there are a significant number of minority adolescents who want to become mothers due to its social status and positive connotations. Preventive efforts need to attempt to convince these females that it is preferable to avoid pregnancy when young. To accomplish this difficult task, changes in our social structure and societal values are needed. It would be necessary to introduce other ways of fulfilling psychological and social needs; of gaining love, understanding, and high self-esteem; and of achieving adult status. Currently, low-income women gain status through their men and their children, since motherhood is their primary role. Fundamental changes in the opportunity structure for these women would be needed to attempt to alter these values. One advantage of addressing these issues at a societal and motivational level is that the focus is on improved levels of functioning rather than specifically on limiting sexual behavior, using contraceptives, sex education, and all the controversies surrounding these efforts (Lindemann & Scott, 1981). One important task in taking this approach is to develop the means to identify females who are positively motivated to become pregnant before they actually do so in order for any preventive efforts to be initiated (Association of Junior Leagues, Inc., 1988; Jorgenson, 1981).

The difficulties of making these changes should not be understated. Regardless of socioeconomic class, there is a popular cultural message that for a woman to be complete and satisfied she needs a man. Women today are bombarded with the message that being successful involves having a man. This message is conveyed even in the more modern women's magazines, which contain articles on ways to attract men, understand men, and keep men. Implied behind these ideas is that there are no lengths to which females should not go in order to achieve this status. This message is a step backward from the current thinking that helps women find alternatives to their more traditional roles. The focus that relegates women to existing only for men is troublesome to those working to prevent premarital adolescent pregnancies.

Findings indicate that those adolescent couples who hold values that support a traditional sex-role structure, in which men tend to dominate, are more likely to be sexually precocious and to be ineffective or inconsistent users of contraceptives. It is suggested that confrontation regarding these sex-role perceptions can help alter them and that it is important to teach children and adolescents to view females as competent and assertive in their relationships. One way to focus on this is to include both partners in sex education classes and to work with them as a couple, so that the decision to delay intercourse can be agreed upon by both without fear of losing the relationship (Jorgenson, 1981).

There is evidence that support from their boyfriends has a positive effect on adolescent females' use of contraceptives. It is suggested that this may be due either to males placing the responsibility for contraception on their girlfriends or to their facilitating rational decision-making and helping their girlfriends face the risk of pregnancy. In a more general way, boyfriends appear to support girlfriends in making decisions, only one of which is regarding contraception. While the role of males has often been assumed to be coercive, exploitive, or else ignored, these findings suggest harnessing males for a greater role in taking responsibility for the use of birth control (Kastner, 1984). It has been suggested that it may be useful to educate teenage boys about their responsibilities regarding sexuality and contraception, while also strengthening sanctions against fathers who decline monetary or emotional involvement with their offspring (Kisker, 1985). Additional support for the potential involvement of males in supporting contraceptive efforts comes from findings of school-based family planning clinics that males make as much use of these services as females (Zabin et al., 1986a).

The need for teen pregnancy prevention efforts directed at males is supported by findings that the attitudes of a group of black males in junior and senior high schools in Baltimore toward sexuality may be conducive to out-of-wedlock conception (Clark, Zabin, & Hardy, 1984). Although 90% of these males reported a recognition of shared responsibility for preventing pregnancy, over half reported that they would engage in unprotected sexual intercourse. While most reported a wish to delay parenthood until their early 20s, they also reported a mean age of commencing intercourse 6 years earlier than the best age to become a parent, which is in turn 2 years earlier than the best age to get married. In addition, while 34% acknowledged that they would be very upset if they got a female pregnant within the next 6 months, 12% reported that they would be happy, and 13% would not be upset. This is even though the majority acknowledge that being a father while still in school would be a problem for them as well as for the mother and child.

Another potential source of support for adolescent females regarding sexual decisions is their parents. However, parents in the United States appear to have a difficult time dealing with and affecting this area of functioning. For example, one study found no relationship between parents' attitudes about premarital sex, or parent-child discussions about sex, and adolescent sexual activity or birth control use (Newcomer & Udry, 1985). In addition, teens' perceptions of their parents' beliefs do not tend to match their parents' actual beliefs. The two relations that did exist— that girls whose mothers report discussing sex with them were less likely to initiate coitus and that girls who report that their mothers discuss birth control with them were more likely to use effective contraceptives—disappeared if it was the other who reported the conversation. It is suggested that the lack of influence of these discussions on child behaviors may be due to the type of conversation held, that although some mothers may be open regarding sexuality in a general way, what may be needed are specific discussions regarding their children's behavior.

However, Kastner (1984) found that while positive and open discussion by parents with daughters has no relation to initiation of sexual activity, it is a strong predictor of contraceptive use once girls do engage in sexual relations. This is interpreted to mean that frank discussion helps female adolescents accept their sexuality and avoid the denial and conflicts that may delay contraceptive use. One problem with this is that mothers generally do not take on this task, so relatively few actually discuss sex with their daughters.

Several potential solutions to this dilemma emerge in the literature, such as including parents in the sex education programs their children attend. This can help promote increased knowledge among parents regarding sexuality and birth control methods, teach them effective means of communicating with their children regarding sexuality, and allow them to reinforce the information learned by their children in the courses (Jorgenson, 1981). It has also been suggested that since parents may not be able to effectively carry birth control information to their children, due to their own embarrassment, the government take over this role. For example, flyers can be developed for parents to give to their adolescents or parents could be encouraged to have their children discuss sex with their physicians (Kisker, 1985).

A different picture emerges regarding cultural and parental attitudes toward teenage sexuality in Sweden, which can serve as a comparison to U.S. views (Brown, 1983). In Sweden a large majority of female teens discuss birth control with their mothers before obtaining it. Parents are more accepting of their children's rights to make decisions, while not necessarily being in favor of premarital sexual relations themselves. Overall, there is strong ideological support for responsible sexual decisions by males and females, for the need to integrate contraceptive education into the wider context of human relationships, and a cultural acceptance of sexuality as part of intimate relationships. While the average age for initiating sexual activity in the United States and Sweden is about the same, the use of birth control is much more widespread in Sweden. Other hypothesized reasons for the increased use of birth control and a decline in adolescent pregnancy in Sweden include a close relationship between schools and family planning services; easy access to contraceptive services, which are free and available without parental consent; and politically secure legislation regarding abortion and contraceptive services that makes them legally and easily available. Sweden was one of the first countries to legalize abortion, although Swedes stress the need for contraceptive services to decrease the need for abortion. Funds are available for various preventive strategies, including government subsidies for contraceptives and training of nurse-midwives to deliver family planning services. One relevant point, however, is that the areas of Sweden with the highest youth unemployment rates also have the highest rates of adolescent fertility. This supports the notion, thought applicable to the lower socioeconomic classes in the United States, that parenthood becomes a career of sorts when there are few other options.

A central focus of Sweden's views of adolescent sexuality is responsibility, which is an area that can be expanded on in U.S. sex education programs. This suggests a shift away from only knowledge regarding sexual behavior, reproduction, and contraception into the area of motivational factors that appear to influence birth control use and sexual risk-taking behavior. One of the central ideas within each of the models to be discussed is that sexuality is a normal part of development, with questions that will be faced by all adolescents (Schinke, 1982; Tauer, 1983). Therefore, making responsible decisions becomes important. Several different programs have been described in the literature, each with a somewhat different perspective, but focusing on values clarification, decision-making, and cognitive skills building, as they may promote increased responsibility toward sexuality and contraception.

One clever preventive idea that has begun to be employed as a school assignment involves caring for "eggbies." Adolescents carry around an egg for a week, caring for it around the clock as if it were an infant. The goal is to gain a sense of the care and responsibility involved in caring for an infant. Students keep journal records of their experiences, which are used as the source of discussions about parental responsibilities (Irwin, 1986).

Tauer (1983) focuses on the necessity of values clarification before effective decision-making can be undertaken. She cites the confusion created by the difference between the moral code passed on by parents and somewhat believed by adolescents that premarital sex is wrong and the fact that teens are thinking about engaging in sexual activity and are surrounded by sexual stimuli by the media and their peers. Values clarification programs are offered to help adolescents understand what they believe in, to determine their own values, and to become more critical of their own thinking and judgments. The values clarification exercises involve bringing preferences and attitudes out into the open, with a goal of bringing values, beliefs, and behaviors into congruence. Exercises involve rating of preferences, agreeing or disagreeing with statements, and discussing what to do about competing alternatives, all relating to sexuality. These values are then used in decision-making processes. The exercises can be done individually, in groups, with a peer or buddy, or even with a same-sex parent. One strategy suggested is to write down potential solutions to help them become more concrete.

Maskay and Juhasz (1983) outline a detailed decision-making process model geared toward helping early adolescents with average-to-low cognitive ability become better at making decisions regarding sexuality. It consists of a series of questions to be considered by the adolescent, beginning with the decision whether to engage in sexual intercourse or abstain and then proceeding with the next logical questions regarding potential consequences—that is, whether to have children; whether to use contraceptives; if pregnant, whether to bear the child; if giving birth, whether to keep the baby or put it up for adoption; and whether to marry or remain single. For each question the adolescents are led through a series of problem-solving processes and must examine the events that made the decision necessary and the available alternative choices of action. Responsible sexual behavior and positive self-esteem are two desired outcomes of the decision-making process and are emphasized as goals. This model is designed to be used with grade school students as well as older adolescents, and, although it requires some training on the part of the teachers, it is rather simple. It is geared toward giving the adolescents a feeling of being in control and removing the irrational, chance probability approach to birth control. Beginning implementation appears successful, although actual evaluation was not reported.

Schinke (1982) describes a school-based model for developing better communication skills, combined with knowledge and behavioral practice. Groups led by school social workers and composed of 12 to 18 students met once or twice weekly for hour-long sessions. Basic information regarding human sexuality, reproduction, and contraception were combined with homework assignments to contact local agencies regarding their services. Group discussions focused on problems related to sexuality, dating, and birth control, with a format of clearly identifying problems and going through a decision-making process of generating multiple solutions, evaluating possible outcomes, developing a plan of action, and practicing implementation in the group session. Demonstration by the leaders and role-play rehearsal with peers as models offered instruction, feedback, practice, and reinforcement. Homework assignments to specifically implement the decisions at which they arrived in class in interactions with others provided further practice and became the focus of discussion for later meetings. The group, run in an urban high school, showed positive results at 6-month follow-up. More responsible sexual behavior was found: fewer instances of intercourse without birth control, more birth control use, and greater commitment to delaying pregnancy.

Another program (Howard, 1985) focused mainly on helping teens become more aware of and learn how to handle pressures from peers to engage in sexual activity. An assumption of this model was that the teens really do not want to engage in sexual behavior but feel pressured to do so. Students learned and practiced ways of noticing and resisting such pressure. Since adolescents tend to respond well to information from peers, the program used slightly older teens in role plays. In addition, there was a component for parents to help them better understand peer pressure and help reinforce the information given in the program.

Another type of cognitive approach was used in one of the few experimental outcome studies in this area (Gerrard et al., 1983). Female undergraduates participated in the study to assess the impact of two preventive interventions and to test the notion that cognitions are important variables in contraceptive behavior. The experimental treatment included cognitive restructuring of attitudes and beliefs regarding birth control. These groups were also compared to a no-treatment control. The focus of the cognitive restructuring program was to challenge common negative attitudes, misconceptions, and beliefs, while increasing positive and realistic thinking regarding birth control. Both the information-only and the cognitive restructuring programs decreased the number of negative beliefs and increased the influence of positive beliefs, an effect that remained at 1-month follow-up. However, at 3-month follow-up only the cognitive restructuring group continued to maintain these new beliefs. Although these groups were run with college students as opposed to younger adolescents, the findings offer preliminary support for the cognitive model. It suggests that a preventive intervention for contraceptive risk-takers can be successful in reducing negative thoughts and irrational beliefs about birth control and in increasing the use of reliable birth control.

In summary, there are numerous areas of concern regarding adolescent sexual behavior as well as many potential areas at which to focus preventive efforts. To limit the focus to only one level of inquiry would ignore other salient factors that are likely to affect sexual decision-making and contraceptive behavior. Major long-term decreases in this country's adolescent pregnancy rate will require changes in knowledge, attitudes, and motivations. Sociocultural changes would need to be involved that offered expanded opportunities and hopes for achievement in adolescents currently living in poverty and changes in the sex-role structure to allow these females to gain higher status in their own right rather than as mothers, wives, or lovers. In addition, greater societal acceptance that adolescents are sexual is more likely to foster more rational decision-making than it is to promote further sexual activity. Regardless, a shift away from the current state of affairs in which adolescents are told by their parents that sex is bad and by the media that it is glamorous will lessen the confusion that likely inhibits effective contraceptive behavior. On a practical note, there is strong evidence that intervention at early ages, even before junior high school, is warranted and that factual information combined with easy accessibility to family planning services increases use of contraceptives. In developing these educational and health-related services it is important to keep in mind adolescents' level of cognitive development and their emotional needs. It is hoped that efforts and funding continue toward primary prevention in this area, as they have the potential to radically improve the lives of substantial numbers of our nation's youth.

References

Abernethy, V., Robbins, D., Abernethy, G. L., Grunebaum, H., & Weiss, J. L. (1975). Identifying women at risk for unwanted pregnancy. *American Journal of Psychiatry, 132*, 1027–1030.

Adams, J. B., & Hatcher, R. A. (1977, March). The perplexing problems of teenage pregnancies. *Urban Health*, 26–49.

Ainsworth, M. D. S., Blehar, M., Waters, E., & Wall, S. (1978). *Patterns of attachment: Observations in the strange situation at home*. Hillsdale, NJ: Lawrence Erlbaum Associates.

Akpom, C. A., Akpom, D., & Davis, M. (1976). Prior sexual behavior of teenagers attending rap sessions for the first time. *Family Planning Perspectives, 8*, 203–208.

Alan Guttmacher Institute. (1976). *11 million teenagers*. New York: New York Planned Parenthood Federation of America.

Alan Guttmacher Institute. (1986). *Teenage pregnancy in industrialized countries: A study*. New Haven: Yale University Press.

Allen-Meares, P. (1984). Adolescent pregnancy and parenting: The forgotten adolescent father and his parents. *Journal of Social Work & Human Sexuality, 3*(1), 27–38.

Als, H., Tronick, E., & Lester, B. (1977). The Brazelton Neonatal Behavioral Assessment Scale (BNBAS). *Journal of Abnormal Child Psychology, 5*, 214–231.

Anderson, B. (1987). Education: Key to minorities gaining jobs. *Black Enterprise, 17*, 45.

Anderson, S. C., & Lauderdale, M. L. (1982). Characteristics of abusive parents: A look at self-esteem. *Child Abuse and Neglect, 6*(3), 285–293.

Arafat, I., & Yorburg, B. (1973). Drug use and the sexual behavior of college women. *Journal of Sex Research, 9*, 21–29.

Archer, R. P. (1987). *Using the MMPI with adolescents*. Hillsdale, NJ: Lawrence Erlbaum Associates.

Archer, R. P., White, J. L., & Orvin, G. H. (1979). MMPI characteristics and correlates among adolescent psychiatric inpatients. *Journal of Clinical Psychology, 35*, 498–504.

Association of Junior Leagues, Inc. (1988). *Where a woman can change the world* (Annual Rep., 1987–88). New York: Author.

Atkinson, K. N. (1986). National programs to promote youth training. *Long Range Planning, 18*, 26.

Atkinson, A. K., & Rickel, A. U. (1984). Postpartum depression in primiparous parents. *Journal of Abnormal Psychology, 93*, 115–119.

Atlas, J., & Rickel, A. U. (1988). Maternal coping styles and adjustment in children. *Journal of Primary Prevention, 8*, 169–185.

Authier, K., & Authier, J. (1982). Intervention with families of pregnant adolescents. In I. Stuart & C. Wells (Eds.), *Pregnancy in adolescence*. New York: Van Nostrand.

Babikian, H. M. & Goldman, A. (1971). A study in teen-age pregnancy. *American Journal of Psychiatry, 128*(6), 111–116.

Baldwin, W. H. (1982). Trends in adolescent contraception, pregnancy and childbearing. In E. R. McAnorey (Ed.), *Premature adolescent pregnancy and parenthood*. New York: Grune & Stratton.

Baldwin, W., & Cain, V. (1980). The children of teenage parents. *Family Planning Perspectives, 12*, 34–43.

Baldwin, J. A., & Oliver, J. E. (1975). Epidemiology and family characteristics of severely abused children. *British Journal of Preventive Social Medicine, 29*, 205–221.

Barber, J., Cernetig, M., Geddes, A., Smith, D., Steacy, A., Lord, D., Van Dusen, L., Jones, D., & Lowthor, W. (1986). Parents, jobs, and children. *Maclean's, 99*, 46.

Barth, R. P., & Schinke, S. P. (1983). Coping with daily strain among pregnant and parenting adolescents. *Journal of Social Service Research, 7*(2), 51–63.

Barth, R. P., & Schinke, S. P. (1984). Enhancing the social supports of teenage mothers. *Social Casework, 65*(9), 523–531.

Barth, R. P., Schinke, S. P., & Maxwell, J. S. (1983). Psychological correlates of teenage motherhood. *Journal of Youth and Adolescence, 12*(6), 471–487.

Bell, R., & Chaskes, J. (1970). Premarital sexual experience among coeds, 1958 and 1968. *Journal of Marriage and Family, 32*, 81–84.

Bierman, B. R., & Streett, R. (1982). Adolescent girls as mothers: Problems in parenting. In I. R. Stuart & C. F. Wells (Eds.), *Pregnancy in adolescence: Needs, problems, and management.* New York: Van Nostrand Reinhold.

Birch, H., & Gussow, G. D. (1970). *Disadvantaged children.* New York: Grune & Stratton.

Black, C. (1979). *It will never happen to me.* New York: Harcourt Brace Jovanovich.

Bloch, D. (1972). Sex education practices of mothers. *Journal of Sex Education and Therapy, 7,* 1–18.

Block, J. (1965). *The child rearing practices report.* Berkeley: University of California, Institute of Human Development.

Blum, B. (1984). Helping teenage mothers. *Public Welfare, 42,* 17–21.

Bolton, F. G. (1980). *The pregnant adolescent: Problems of premature adulthood.* Beverly Hills: Sage.

Bracken, M., Klerman, L., & Bracken, M. (1978). Abortion, adoption, or motherhood: An empirical study of decision making during pregnancy. *American Journal of Obstetrics and Gynecology, 130*(3), 251–262.

Brenner, A. (1985). Wednesday's child; in the outcry over physical and sexual abuse, the plight of more than a million neglected children has been virtually ignored. *Psychology Today, 19,* 45–46.

Broussard, E. R. (1982). Primary prevention of psychosocial disorders. Assessment of outcome. In L. A. Bond & J. M. Joffe (Eds.), *Facilitating infant and early childhood development.* Hanover, NH: University Press of New England.

Broussard, E. R., & Hartner, M. S. (1971). Further considerations regarding maternal perceptions of the first born. In J. Hellmuth (Ed.), *Exceptional infant, Vol. 2: Studies in abnormalities.* New York: Brunner Mazel.

Brown, H., Adams, R. G., & Kellam, S. G., (1981). A longitudinal study of teenage motherhood and symptoms of distress: The Woodlawn Community Epidemiological Project. In R. Simmons (Ed.), *Research in community mental health* (Vol. 2). Greenwich, CT: JAI Press.

Brown, P. (1983). The Swedish approach to sex education and adolescent pregnancy: Some impressions. *Family Planning Perspectives, 15,* 90–95.

Brown, S., Lieberman, J., & Miller, W. (1975). *Young adults as partners and planners: A preliminary report on the antecedents of responsible family formation.* Paper presented at 103rd Annual Meeting of the American Public Health Association, Chicago.

Buchholz, E. S., & Gol, B. (1986). More than playing house: A developmental perspective on the strengths in teenage motherhood. *American Journal of Orthopsychiatry, 56*(3), 347–359.

Burgess, E., & Wallin P. (1953). *Engagement and marriage.* New York: Lippincott.

Butler, C. (1989). *Social support and childrearing practices of teenage mothers.* Unpublished master's thesis, Wayne State University, Detroit.

Butler, O. B. (1986). The young worker; why Johnny can't get a job. *Current,* 19.

Camp, B. W., & Morgan, L. J. (1984). Child-rearing attitudes and personality characteristics in adolescent mothers: Attitudes toward the infant. *Journal of Pediatric Psychology, 9,* 57–64.

Campbell, M. (1987, May). *Overview of the teen parent initiative.* Paper presented at the First Biennial Conference on Community Research and Action, Columbia, SC.

Cannon-Bonventre, K. (1979). *The ecology of help-seeking behavior among adolescent parents*. Cambridge, MA: American Institutes for Research.

Carey, S. E. (1981). *Maturation and the development of spatial ability in children.* Paper presented at the conference Gender Role Development: Conceptual and Methodological Issues, National Institutes of Health, Bethesda, MD.

Carey, S. E., & Diamond, R. (1980). Maturational determination of the developmental course of face encoding. In D. Caplan (Ed.), *Biological studies of mental processes*. Cambridge: MIT Press.

Carey, S. E., Diamond, R., & Woods, B. (1980). Development of face recognition—A maturational component? *Developmental Psychology, 16*, 257–269.

Carlson, M. L., Kaiser, K. L., Yeaworth, R. C., & Carlson, R. E. (1984). An exploratory study of life-change events, social support and pregnancy decisions in adolescents. *Adolescence, 19*, 765–780.

Carlson, E., & Stinson, K. (1982). Motherhood, marriage timing and marital stability: A research report. *Social Forces, 61*(1), 258–267.

Carpenter, T. G. (1985). The new anti-youth movement. [Current legislation is taking away the rights of teenagers]. *Nation, 240*, 39.

Centers for Disease Control. (1978, April). *Abortion surveillance, 1976*. Atlanta: DHEW Public Health Services.

Center for Population Research. (1983). *National Institute of Health and Human Development. Progress Report*. Bethesda, MD: Author.

Chesler, J. S., & Davis, S. A. (1980). Problem pregnancy and abortion counseling with teenagers. *Social Casework, 61*, 173–179.

Chilman, C. (1963). *The educational-vocational aspirations and behaviors of unmarried and married undergraduates at Syracuse University*. Unpublished manuscript.

Chilman, C. (1979). *Adolescent sexuality in a changing American society: Social and psychological perspectives*. Washington, DC: U. S. Government Printing Office.

Chilman, C. (1983). *Adolescent sexuality in a changing society* (2nd ed.). New York: Wiley.

Chilman, C. (1986). Some psychosocial aspects of adolescent sexual and contraceptive behaviors in a changing American society. In J. Lancaster & B. Hamburg (Eds.), *School-age pregnancy and parenthood* (pp. 191–217). New York: Aldine DeGruyter.

Christensen, H., & Gregg, C. (1970). Changing sex norms in America and Scandinavia. *Journal of Marriage and the Family, 32*, 616–627.

Clark, S. D., Zabin, L. S., & Hardy, J. B. (1984). Sex, contraception and parenthood: Experience and attitudes among urban black young men. *Family Planning Perspectives, 16*, 77–82.

Clausen, J. A. (1975). The social meaning of differential physical and sexual maturation. In S. E. Dragastin & G. H. Elder (Eds.), *Adolescence in the life cycle: Psychological change and social context*. Washington, DC: Hemisphere.

Cochrane, R., & Robertson, A. (1973). The life events inventory: A measure of the relative severity of psychosocial stressors. *Journal of Psychosomatic Research, 17*, 135–139.

Coleman, J. C. (1980). Friendship and the peer group in adolescence. In J. Adelson (Ed.), *Handbook of adolescent psychology*. New York: Wiley.

Collier, J. L. (1980, February). Abortion: How men feel about it. *Glamour*, p. 165.

Conger, J. J., & Petersen, A. C. (1984). *Adolescence and youth* (3rd ed.). New York: Harper & Row.

Connolly, L. (1975). Little mothers. *Human Behavior, 11*, 17–23.

Costanzo, P. R., & Shaw, M. E. (1966). Conformity as a function of age level. *Child Development, 37*, 967–975.

Crittenden, P. M. (1983). *Maltreated infants: Vulnerability and resilience*. Paper presented at the biennial meeting of the Society for Research in Child Development, Detroit.

Crittenden, P. M., & Snell, M. E. (1983). Intervention to improve mother-infant interaction. *Infant Mental Health Journal, 4*, 23–31.

Croake, J., & James, B. (1973). A four year comparison of premarital sexual attitudes. *Journal of Sex Research, 9*, 91–96.

Cvetkovich, G., Grote, B., Bjorseth, A., & Sarkissian, J. (1975). On the psychology of adolescents' use of contraception. *Journal of Sex Research, 11*, 256–270.

Cvetkovich, G., & Grote, B. (1976, May). Psychological factors associated with adolescent premarital coitus. Paper presented at the National Institute of Child Health and Human Development, Bethesda, MD.

Damon, W., & Hart, D. (1982). The development of self-understanding from infancy through adolescence. *Child Development, 53*, 841–864.

Daniels, S. (1986). Relationship of employment status to mental health and family variables in black men from single-parent families. *Journal of Applied Psychology, 71*, 386.

Darney, P. (1976). Postabortion and postpartum contraceptive acceptance among adolescents. Paper presented at the annual meeting of the American Public Health Association, Miami Beach, FL.

Dawson, D. A. (1986). The effects of sex education on adolescent behavior. *Family Planning Perspectives, 18*, 162–170.

de Anda, D. (1984). Informal support networks of Hispanic mothers: A comparison across age groups. *Journal of Social Service Research, 7*(3), 89–105.

DeLameter, J., & MacCorquodale, M. (1979). *Premarital sexuality: Attitudes, relationships, behaviors*. Madison: University of Wisconsin Press.

Delatte, J. G., Orgeron, K., Preis, J. (1985). Project Scan: Counseling teen-age parents in a school setting. *Journal of School Health, 55*(1), 24–26.

Dohwenrend, B. S., & Dohwenrend, B. P. (1974). *Stressful life events: Their nature and effects*. New York: Wiley.

Donovan, R., Hawkins, A., Hatch, O. G., Clay, W., Dixon, J. C., Tucker, W., Donison, R., Welch, F., & O'Hara, J. G. (1985). Should Congress enact proposed subminimum wage legislation for youth? *Congressional Digest, 64*, 106.

Dreyer, P. H. (1982). Sexuality during adolescence. In B. Wolman (Ed.), *Handbook of developmental psychology* (pp. 559–601). Englewood Cliffs, NJ: Prentice-Hall.

Dreyfuss, S. (1985). A different kind of schooling [Lents Education Center in Portland]. *Progressive, 49*, 19.

Drotar, D., Malone, C. A., Negray, J., & Dennstedt, M. (1981). Psychosocial assessment and care for infants hospitalized for nonorganic failure to thrive. *Journal of Clinical Child Psychology, 10*, 63–66.

Dryfoos, J. (1985). School-based health clinics: A new approach to preventing adolescent pregnancy? *Family Planning Perspectives, 17*, 70–75.

Edwards, L. E., Steinman, K. A., Arnold, K. A., Hakanson, E. Y. (1980). Adolescent pregnancy prevention services in high school clinics. *Family Planning Perspectives, 12*, 6–14.

Egeland, B., Breitenbucher, M., & Rosenberg, D. (1980). Prospective study of the significance of life stress in the etiology of child abuse. *Journal of Consulting and Clinical Psychology, 48*, 195–205.

Egeland, B., & Brunquell, D. (1979). An at-risk approach to the study of child abuse: Some preliminary findings. *Journal of the American Academy of Child Psychiatry, 18*, 219–235.

Ehrenworth, N. V., & Archer, R. P. (1985). A comparison of clinical accuracy ratings of interpretive approaches for adolescent MMPI responses. *Journal of Personality Assessment, 49*, 413–421.

Ehrmann, W. (1959). *Premarital dating behavior.* New York: Holt, Rinehart & Winston.

Elkind, D. (1967). Egocentrism in adolescence. *Child Development, 38*, 1025–1034.

Elkind, D. (1984). *All grown up and no place to go: Teenagers in crisis.* New York: Addison-Wesley.

Erikson, E. H. (1959). The problem of ego identity. *Psychological Issues, 1*(1), 101–164.

Evans, J., Selstad, G., & Welcher, W. (1976). Teenagers: Fertility control behavior and attitudes before and after abortion, childbearing, or negative pregnancy test. *Family Planning Perspectives, 8*, 192–200.

Eversoll, D. (1979). The changing father role: Implications for parent education programs for today's youth. *Adolescence, 14*(55), 535–544.

Faigel, H. C. (1967). Unwed pregnant adolescents—A synthesis of current viewpoints. *Clinical Pediatrics, 6*, 281–285.

Falkenberg, J. (1985). Teen pregnancy: Who opts for adoption? *Psychology Today, 19*, 16.

Feather, N. T., & O'Brien, G. E. (1986). A longitudinal study of the effects of employment and unemployment on school-leavers. *Journal of Occupational Psychology, 59*, 121.

Feldman, H. (1977). *Cornell studies of marital development: Study in the transition to parenthood.* Ann Arbor: University Microfilms International.

Ferrell, M., Tolone, W., & Walsh, R. (1977). Maturational and societal changes in the sexual double standard. *Journal of Marriage and the Family, 39*, 225–271.

Field, T. (1980). Interactions of preterm and term infants with their lower- and middle-class teenage and adult mothers. In T. M. Field, S. Goldberg, D.

Stern, & A. M. Sosteck (Eds.), *High-risk infants and children: Adult and peer interactions*. New York: Academic Press.

Field, T. M. (1982). Infants born at risk: Early compensatory experiences. In L. A. Bond & J. M. Joffe (Eds.), *Facilitating infant and early childhood development*. Hanover, NH: University Press of New England.

Finkel, M., & Finkel, D. (1975). Sexual contraceptive knowledge, attitudes and behaviors of male adolescents. *Family Planning Perspectives, 7*, 256–260.

Fine, P., & Pape, M. (1982). Pregnant teenagers in need of social networks: Diagnostic parameters. In I. R. Stewart and C. F. Wells (Eds.), *Pregnancy in adolescence: Needs, problems, and management*. New York: Van Nostrand Reinhold.

Flaherty, E., Maracek, J., Olssen, K., & Wilcove, G. (1982). *Psychological factors associated with fertility regulation among adolescents* (Final Report. Contract No. N01-HD-82883-NICHHD). Bethesda, MD: National Institute of Child Health and Human Development.

Ford Foundation Report. (1983). *Child survival/fair start*. New York: Author.

Forrest, J., Sullivan, E., & Tietze, C. (1979). Abortion in the United States. *Family Planning Perspectives, 11*, 329–341.

Fox, G. L. (1979, May–June). The family's influence in adolescent sexual behavior. *Children Today*, pp. 21–36.

Fox, G., & Inazu, J. (1980). Patterns and outcomes of mother-daughter communication about sexuality. *Journal of Social Issues, 36*, 7–29.

Freeman, E. W., Rickels, K., Mudd, E. B., & Huggins, G. R. (1982). Never-pregnant adolescents and family planning programs: Contraception, continuation, and pregnancy risk. *American Journal of Public Health, 72*, 815–822.

Furstenberg, F. F. (1980). Burdens and benefits: The impact of early childbearing on the family. *Journal of Social Issues, 36*(1), 64–87.

Furstenberg, F. F., Jr. (1976). *Unplanned parenthood: The social consequences of teenage child bearing*. New York: Free Press.

Furstenberg, F. F., Jr. (1980). The impact of early childbearing on the family. *Journal of Social Issues, 36*, 64–87.

Furstenberg, F. F., Jr. (1981). Implicating the family. Teenage parenthood and kinship involvement. In T. Ooms (Ed.), *Teenage pregnancy in a family context—implications for policy*. Philadelphia: Temple University Press.

Furstenberg, F., & Crawford, A. (1978). Family support: Helping teenage mothers to cope. *Family Planning Perspectives, 10*, 322–333.

Gabrielson, I., Klerman, L., Currie, J., Tyler, N., & Jekel, J. (1970). Suicide attempts in a population pregnant as teen-agers. *American Journal of Public Health, 60*, 2289–2301.

Garbarino, J. (1976). A preliminary study of some ecological correlates of child abuse: The impact of socioeconomic stress on mothers. *Child Development, 47*, 178–185.

Gebhard, P., Pomeroy, W., Martin, C., & Christensen, C. (1956). *Pregnancy, birth, and abortion*. New York: Harper and Brothers.

Gerrard, M. (1987). Sex, sex guilt, and contraceptive use revisited: The 1980's. *Journal of Personality and Social Psychology, 52*, 975–980.

Gerrard, M., McCann, L., & Fortini, M. (1983). Prevention of unwanted pregnancy. *American Journal of Community Psychology, 11*, 153–167.

Gil, D. (1970). *Violence against children.* Cambridge, MA: Harvard University Press.

Glenn, N., & Weaver, C. (1979). Attitudes towards premarital, extramarital and homosexual relations in the U. S. in the 1970's. *Journal of Sex Research, 15*, 108–118.

Goldberg, S. (1979). Premature birth: Consequences for the parent-infant relationship. *American Scientist, 67*, 214–220.

Goldsmith, S., Gabrielson, M., & Gabrielson, I. (1972). Teenagers, sex and contraception. *Family Planning Perspectives, 4*, 32–38.

Goldfarb, J. L., Mumford, D. M., Shurn, D. A., Smith, P. B., Flowers, C., & Shum, C. (1977). An attempt to detect "pregnancy susceptibility" in indigent adolescent girls. *Journal of Youth and Adolescence, 6*, 127–144.

Goode, W. J. (1961). Illegitimacy, anomie, and cultural penetration. *American Sociological Review, 26*, 910–925.

Gorlor, E. R., Jr. (1986). Teaching young teenagers skills for adolescence. *Education Digest, 52*, 36.

Graves, W. (1976, April). *Sequelae of unwanted pregnancy. A comparison of unmarried abortion and maternity patients.* Paper presented at the Population Association of America, Montreal, Canada.

Greer, J. G. (1982). Adoptive placement: Developmental and psychotherapeutic issues. In I. R. Stuart and C. F. Wells (Eds.), *Pregnancy in adolescence.* New York: Van Nostrand Reinhold.

Guttentag, M., Salasin, S., & Belle, D. (1980). *The mental health of women.* New York: Academic Press.

Hale, D. (1986). Alagasoe assists its community; innovative community service program aids disadvantaged youth, low-income families [Alabama Gas Co.]. *Pipeline & Gas Journal, 213*, 12.

Hamburg, B. (1986). Subsets of adolescent mothers: Developmental, biomedical, and psychosocial issues. In J. Lancaster & B. Hamburg (Eds.), *School-age pregnancy and parenthood.* New York: Aldine de Gruyter.

Harlap, S., Shiono, P., Ramcharan, S., et al. (1979). A prospective study of fetal losses after induced abortions. *New England Journal of Medicine, 301*, 677–681.

Harrison, S. S. (1987). Aid for unwed teens. *Black Enterprise, 17*, 17.

Hatcher, S. (1973). The adolescent experience of pregnancy and abortion: A developmental analysis. *Journal of Youth and Adolescence, 2*, 53–102.

Hatcher, S. (1976). Understanding adolescent pregnancy and abortion. *Primary Care, 3*, 407–425.

Hathaway, S. R. (1946). The Multiphasic Personality Inventory. *Modern Hospital, 66*, 65–67.

Heiman, M., & Levitt, E. G. (1960). The role of separation and depression in out-of-wedlock pregnancy. *American Journal of Orthopsychiatry, 30*, 166–174.

Hendricks, L. E. (1983). Suggestions for reaching unmarried black adolescent fathers. *Child Welfare, 62*(2), 141–146.

Hendricks, L. E., & Montgomery, T. (1983). A limited population of unmarried adolescent fathers: A preliminary report on their views on fatherhood and their relationship with the mothers of their children. *Adolescence, 18*(69), 201–210.

Highlee, K. L. (1981). Parents' perceptions of their preschool childrens' obedience. *Psychology Reports, 49*(1), 209–210.

Hogan, D. P., Astone, N. M., & Kitagawa, E. M. (1985). Social and environmental factors influencing contraceptive use among black adolescents. *Family Planning Perspectives, 17*, 165–169.

Hogan, D. P., & Kitagawa, E. M. (1985). The impact of social status, family structure, and neighborhood on the fertility of black adolescents. *American Journal of Sociology, 90*, 825–853.

Holden, C. (1985). Few long-term gains in youth employment project [Youth Employment and Demonstration Projects Act]. *Science, 230*, 1257.

Hooke, J. F., & Marks, P. A. (1962). MMPI characteristics of pregnancy. *Journal of Clinical Psychology, 18*, 316–317.

Horn, J. M., Green, M., Carney, R., & Erickson, M. T. (1975). Bias against genetic hypothesis in adoption studies. *Archives of General Psychiatry, 32*, 1365–1367.

Hornick, J., Doran, L., & Crawford, S. (1979). Premarital contraceptive behaviors among young male and female adolescents. *Family Coordinator, 28*, 181–190.

Howard, M. (1985). Postponing sexual involvement among adolescents. *Journal of Adolescent Health Care, 6*, 271–277.

Howard, M. (1979). *Only human—Teenage pregnancy and parenthood.* New York: Avon Books.

Hunt, M. (1974). *Sexual behaviors in the 1970's.* Chicago: Playboy Press.

Inhelder, B., & Piaget, J. (1958). *The growth of logical thinking from childhood to adolescence.* New York: Basic Books.

Institute of Medicine. (1975). *Legalized abortion and the public health.* Washington, DC: National Academy of Sciences.

Irwin, J. (1986, June 5). Students take a crack at parenthood. *Detroit Free Press,* p. 4A.

Isaacs, C. (1981). A brief review of the characteristics of abuse-prone parents. *Behavior Therapist, 4*(2), 5–8.

Jessor, S., & Jessor, R. (1975). Transition from virginity to nonvirginity among youth: A social-psychological study over time. *Developmental Psychology, 11*, 473–484.

Joffe, C. (1986). *The regulation of sexuality: Experiences of family planning workers.* Philadelphia: Temple University Press.

Johnson, C., Loxterkamp, D., & Albanese, M. (1982). Effect of high school students' knowledge of child development and child health on approaches to child discipline. *Pediatrics, 69*(5), 558–562.

Johnson, K., & Rosenbaum, S. (1986). *Building health programs for teenagers.* Unpublished manuscript, Children's Defense Fund, Washington, DC.

Jones, J. B., Namerow, P. B., & Philliber, S. (1982). Adolescents' use of a hospital-based contraceptive program. *Family Planning Perspectives, 14*, 224–231.

Jones, D. C., Rickel, A. U., & Smith, R. L. (1980). Maternal child rearing practices and social problem solving strategies among preschoolers. *Developmental Psychology, 16*, 241–242.

Jorgenson, S., King, S., and Torrey, B. (1980). Dyadic and social network influencing an adolescent exposure to pregnancy risk. *Journal of Marriage and the Family, 42*, 141–155.

Jorgenson, S. R. (1981). Sex education and the reduction of adolescent pregnancies: Prospects for the 1980's. *Journal of Early Adolescence, 1*, 38–52.

Jorgenson, S. R. (1983). Beyond adolescent pregnancy: Research frontiers for early adolescent sexuality. *Journal of Early Adolescence, 3*, 141–156.

Juhasz, A. M. (1974). The unmarried adolescent parent. *Adolescence, 9*, 263–272.

Justice, B., & Duncan, D. F. (1976). Life crises as a precursor to child abuse. *Public Health Reports, 91*, 110–115.

Kantner, J., & Zelnik, M. (1972). Sexual experiences of young unmarried women in the U. S. *Family Planning Perspectives, 4*, 9–17.

Kaplan, H. B., Smith, P. B., & Pokorny, A. D. (1979). Psychosocial antecedents of unwed motherhood among indigent adolescents. *Journal of Youth and Adolescence, 8*, 181–207.

Kastner, L. S. (1984). Ecological factors predicting adolescent contraceptive use: Implications for prevention. *Journal of Adolescent Health Care, 5*, 79–86.

Kavrell, S. M., & Petersen, A. C. (1984). Patterns of achievement in early adolescence. In M. L. Maehr & M. W. Steinkamp (Eds.), *Women and science.* Greenwich, CT: JAI Press.

Keating, D. P. (1980). Thinking processes in adolescence. In J. Adelson (Ed.), *Handbook of adolescent psychology.* New York: Wiley.

Kessler, R. C., & Cleary, P. D. (1980). Social class and psychological distress. *American Sociological Review, 45*, 463–477.

Kinard, E. M., & Klerman, L. V. (1980). Teenage parenting and child abuse: Are they related? *American Journal of Orthopsychiatry, 50*(3), 481–488.

Kinard, E. M., & Reinherz, H. (1984). Behavioral and emotional functioning in children of adolescent mothers. *American Journal of Orthopsychiatry, 54*(4), 578–594.

King, T., & Fullard, W. (1982). Teenage mothers and their infants: New findings on the home environment. *Journal of Adolescence, 5*(4), 333–346.

Kinsey, A., Pomeroy, W., & Martin, C. (1948). *Sexual behavior in the human male.* Philadelphia: W. B. Saunders.

Kinsey, A., Pomeroy, W., Martin, C., & Gebhard, P. (1953). *Sexual behavior in the human female.* Philadelphia: W. B. Saunders.

Kirby, D., Alter, J., & Scales, P. (1979). *An analysis of United States sex education programs and evaluation methods* (Rep. No. CDC-2021-79-DK-FR). Washington, DC: U.S. Department of Health, Education, and Welfare.

Kisker, E. E. (1984). The effectiveness of family planning clinics in serving adolescents. *Family Planning Perspectives, 16*, 212–218.

Kisker, E. E. (1985). Teenagers talk about sex, pregnancy and contraception. *Family Planning Perspectives, 17*, 83–90.

Klerman, L. (1981). Programs for pregnant adolescents and young parents: Their development and assessment. In K. Scott, T. Field, & Robertson (Eds.), *Teenage parents and their offspring*. New York: Grune & Stratton.

Klerman, L., Bracken, M., Jekel, J., & Bracken, M. (1982). The delivery-abortion decision among adolescents. In I. Stuart & C. Wells (Eds.), *Pregnancy in adolescence*. New York: Van Nostrand Reinhold.

Koff, E., Rierdan, J., and Silverstone, E. (1978). Changes in representation of body image as a function of menarcheal status. *Developmental Psychology, 14*, 635–642.

Komarovsky, M. (1962). *Blue collar marriage*. New York: Random House.

LaBarre, M. (1968). Pregnancy experiences among married adolescents. *American Journal of Orthopsychiatry, 38*, 47–55.

Ladner, J. (1971). *Tomorrow's tomorrow: The black women*. Garden City, NJ: Doubleday.

Lahey, B. B., Conger, R. D., Atkeson, B. M., & Treiber, F. A. (1984). Parenting behavior and emotional status of physically abusive mothers. *Journal of Consulting and Clinical Psychology, 52*, 1062–1071.

Lancaster, J. (1986). Human adolescence and reproduction: An evolutionary perspective. In J. Lancaster & B. Hamburg (Eds.), *School-age pregnancy and parenthood* (pp. 17–37). New York: Aldine de Gruyter.

Landry, E., Bertrand, J. T., Cherry, F., & Rice, J. (1986). Teen pregnancy in New Orleans: Factors that differentiate teens who deliver, abort, and successfully contracept. *Journal of Youth and Adolescence, 15*(3), 259–274.

Landy, S., Schubert, J., Cleland, J. F., Clark, C., & Montgomery, J. (1983). Teenage pregnancy: Family syndrome? *Adolescence, 71*, 679–694.

Landy, S., Schubert, J., Cleland, J. F., & Montgomery, J. S. (1984). The effect of research with teenage mothers on the development of their infants. *Journal of Applied Social Psychology, 14*(5), 461–468.

Landy, S., Cleland, J., & Schubert, J. (1984). The individuality of teenage mothers and its implication for intervention strategies. *Journal of Adolescence, 10*, 7–23.

LaResche, L., Strobino, D., Parks, P., Fischer, P., & Smeriglio, V. (1981). The relationship of observed maternal behavior. TV questionnaire measures of parenting knowledge, attitudes, and emotional state in adolescent mothers. *Journal of Youth and Adolescence, 12*(1), 19–31.

Lewis, A. C. (1985). Young and poor in America [Washington Report]. *Phi Delta Kappan, 67*, 251.

Lewis, C. C. (1980). A comparison of minors' and adults' pregnancy decisions. *American Journal of Orthopsychiatry, 50*(3), 446–453.

Lindemann, C. (1974). *Birth control and unmarried young women*. New York: Springer.

Lindemann, C., & Scott, W. J. (1981). Wanted and unwanted pregnancy in early adolescence: Evidence from a clinic population. *Journal of Early Adolescence, 1*, 185–193.

Loesch, J., & Greenberg, N. (1962). Some specific areas of conflict observed during pregnancy: A contraceptive study of married and unmarried women. *American Journal of Orthopsychiatry, 32*, 624–636.

Loevinger, J. (1979). Construct validity of the Sentence Completion Test of ego development. *Applied Psychological Measurement, 3*, 281–311.

Loevinger, J., & Wessler, R. (1970). *Measuring ego development: Construction and use of a sentence completion test.* San Francisco: Jossey-Bass.

Luker, K. (1975). *Taking chances: Abortion and the decision not to contracept.* Berkeley: University of California Press.

Malmquist, C. P., Kircsuk, T. J., & Spano, R. M. (1967). Mothers with multiple illegitimacies. *Psychiatric Quarterly, 41*, 339–354.

Maracek, J. (1987). Counseling adolescents with problem pregnancies. *American Psychologist, 42*, 89–93.

Marcia, J. E. (1966). Development and validation of ego identity status. *Journal of Personality and Social Psychology, 3*, 551–558.

Marcia, J. E., & Friedman, M. L. (1970). Ego identity status in college women. *Journal of Personality, 2*, 249–263.

Marsiglio, W., & Mott, F. L. (1986). The impact of sex education on sexual activity, contraceptive use and premarital pregnancy among American teenagers. *Family Planning Perspectives, 18*, 151–161.

Maskay, M. H., & Juhasz, A. M. (1983). The decision-making process model: Design and use for adolescent sexual decisions. *Family Relations, 32*, 111–116.

McAdoo, H. P. (1985). Strategies used by black single mothers against stress. Slipping through the cracks: The status of black women. *Review of Black Political Economy, 14*, 153.

McCarthy, B. (1986). Youth employment; for some a most elusive goal. *Nation's Cities Weekly, 9*, 3.

McCarthy, J. D., & Hoge, D. R. (1982). Analysis of age effects in longitudinal studies of adolescent self-esteem. *Developmental Psychology, 18*, 372–379.

McKay, M. J., & Richardson, H. (1973). Personality differences between one-time recidivist unwed mothers. *Journal of Genetic Psychology, 122*, 207–210.

McLanahan, S. S., Wedemeyer, N. V., & Adelberg, T. (1981). Network structure, social support, and psychological well-being in the single-parent family. *Journal of Marriage and the Family, 43*, 601–612.

Mech, E. V. (1986). Pregnant adolescents: Communicating the adoption option. *Child Welfare, 65*, 555–567.

Meyerowitz, J., & Malev, J. (1973). Pubescent attitudinal correlates antecedent to adolescent illegitimate pregnancy. *Journal of Youth and Adolescence, 2*, 251–258.

Miller, S. H. (1984). The relationship between adolescent childbearing and child maltreatment. *Child Welfare, 63*(6), 553–557.

Miller, W. B. (1973). Conception mastery: Ego control of the psychological and behavioral antecedents to conception. *Comments on Contemporary Psychiatry, 1*, 157–177.

Miller, W. (1976, September). *Some psychological factors predictive of undergraduate sexual and contraceptive behaviors.* Paper presented at the 84th Annual Convention of the American Psychological Association, Washington, DC.

Minde, K. K., Shosenberg, N. E., & Marton, P. (1982). The effects of self-help groups in a premature nursery on maternal autonomy and caretaking style 1 year later. In L. A. Bond & J. M. Joffe (Eds.), *Facilitating infant and early childhood development*. Hanover, NH: University Press of New England.

Minde, K., Shosenberg, N., Marton, P., Thompson, J., Ripley, J., & Burns, S. (1980). Self-help groups in a premature nursery: A controlled evaluation. *Journal of Pediatrics, 96*, 933–940.

Minde, K., Shosenberg, N., & Thompson, P. (1983). Self-help groups in a premature nursery: Infant behavior and parental competence 1 year later. In E. Galenson & J. Call (Eds.), *Frontiers of infant psychiatry*. New York: Basic Books.

Mindick, B., & Oskamp, S. (1982). Individual differences among adolescent contraceptors: Some implications for intervention. In I. Stuart & C. Wells (Eds.), *Pregnancy in adolescence* (pp. 140–176). New York: Van Nostrand Reinhold.

Mindick, B., Oskamp, S., & Berger, D. E. (1977). Prediction of success or failure in birth planning: An approach to prevention of individual and family stress. *American Journal of Community Psychology, 5*, 447–459.

Moore, K., & Caldwell, S. (1977). *Out of wedlock childbearing*. Washington, DC: The Urban Institute.

Morse, C., Sahler, O., & Friedman, S. A. (1970). A three-year follow-up study of abused and neglected children. *American Journal of Diseases of Children, 120*, 439–446.

Mott, F. L. (1986). The pace of repeated childbearing among young American mothers. *Family Planning Perspectives, 18*, 5–12.

Moyer, L. S., & de Rosenroll, D. A. (1984). Goal attainment scaling: Its use with pregnant and single-parent teenagers in an alternative education setting. *Canadian Counsellor, 18*(3), 111–116.

Nelson, W. (1986). MMPI personality differences in various populations of the unwed mother. *Journal of Clinical Psychology, 42*(1), 114–119.

Nelson, W., Gumlak, J., & Politano, P. (1986). MMPI personality differences in various populations of the unwed mother. *Journal of Clinical Psychology, 42*(1), 114–119.

Newcomer, S. F., & Udry, J. R. (1985). Parent-child communication and adolescent sexual behavior. *Family Planning Perspectives, 17*(4), 169–174.

Newman, B. M., & Newman, P. R. (1975). *Development through life: A psychosocial approach*. Homewood, IL: Dorsey Press.

Nilson, D. M. (1985). The youngest workers: 14- and 15-year-olds. *Education Digest, 51*, 53.

Olson, L. (1980). Social and psychological correlates of pregnancy resolution among adolescent women: A review. *American Journal of Orthopsychiatry, 50*, 432–445.

Olson, R. J., Smith, D. A., Farkas, G. (1986). Structural and reduced-form models of choice among alternatives in continuous time: Youth employment under a guaranteed jobs program. *Econometrics, 54*, 375.

O'Malley, P. M., & Bachman, J. G. (1983). Self-esteem: Change and stability between ages 13 and 23. *Developmental Psychology, 19*, 257–268.

One day at a time in Al-Anon. (1985). New York: Al-Anon Family Group Headquarters.

Oritt, E., Paul, S., & Behrmann, J. (1985). The perceived support network inventory. *American Journal of Community Psychology, 13*(5), 565–582.

Packard, V. (1968). *The sexual wilderness.* New York: David McKay.

Paffenberger, R. S., & McCabe, L. J. (1966). The effect of obstetric and perinatal events on rise of mental illness in women of child bearing age. *American Journal of Public Health, 56,* 400–407.

Parmelee, A. H., & Haber, A. (1973). Who is the "risk infant"? In H. J. Osofsky (Ed.), *Clinical obstetrics and gynecology.* New York: Harper & Row.

Pasamanick, B., & Knobloch, H. (1961). Epidemiologic studies on the complications of pregnancy and the birth process. In G. Caplan (Ed.), *Prevention of mental disorders in children.* New York: Basic Books.

Perez-Reyes, M., & Falk, R. (1973). Follow-up after therapeutic abortion in early adolescence. *Archives of General Psychiatry, 28,* 120–126.

Pestrak, V. A., & Martin, D. (1985). Cognitive development and aspects of adolescent sexuality. *Adolescence, 20,* 981–987.

Petersen, A. C. (1983). Pubertal change and cognition. In J. Brooks-Gunn & A. C. Petersen (Eds.), *Girls at puberty: Biological and psychosocial perspectives.* New York: Plenum Press.

Petersen, A. C., & Crockett, L. (1986). Pubertal development and its relation to cognitive and psychosocial development in adolescent girls: Implications for parenting. In J. Lancaster & B. Hamburg (Eds.), *School-age pregnancy and parenthood* (pp. 147–175). New York: Aldine de Gruyter.

Piaget, J. (1972). Intellectual evolution from adolescence to adulthood. *Human Development, 15,* 1–12.

Pitt, B. (1968). "A typical" depression following childbirth. *British Journal of Psychiatry, 114,* 1325–1335.

Planned Parenthood Federation of America. (1985). *Fact sheet: Teenagers, sexuality education, birth control and pregnancy: National overview (1984/5).* New York: Author.

Polit, D. F. (1987). Routes to self-sufficiency: Teenage mothers and employment. *Children Today, 16,* 6.

Polit, D. F., & Kahn, J. R. (1985). Project Redirection: Evaluation of a comprehensive program for disadvantaged teenage mothers. *Family Planning Perspectives, 17,* 150–155.

Pope, H. (1967). Unwed mothers and their sex partners. *Journal of Marriage and the Family, 29,* 555–567.

Presser, H. (1977). Guessing and misinformation about pregnancy risks among urban mothers. *Family Planning Perspectives, 9,* 234–236.

Presser, H. (1978). Age at menarche, socio-sexual behavior and fertility. *Social Biology, 2,* 94–101.

Quinlen, A. (1987). Baby craving. *Life, 10*(6), 23–26.

Rader, G. E., Bekker, L.D., Broun, L., & Richardt, C. (1978). Psychological correlates of unwanted pregnancy. *Journal of Abnormal Psychology, 87,* 373–376.

Radloff, L. S., & Rae, D. S. (1979). Susceptibility and precipitating factors in depression: Sex differences and similarities. *Journal of Abnormal Psychology, 88,* 174–181.

Rains, P. (1971). *Becoming an unwed mother—a sociological account.* Chicago: Aldine de Gruyter.

Rainwater, L. (1970). *Behind ghetto walls: Black families in a federal slum.* Chicago: Aldine de Gruyter.

Ralph, N., & Edgington, A. (1983). An evaluation of an adolescent family planning program. *Journal of Adolescent Health Care, 4,* 158–162.

Ralph, N., Lochman, J., & Thomas, M. (1984). Psychosocial characteristics of pregnant and nulliparous adolescents. *Adolescence, 19*(74), 283–294.

Ramey, C. T., & Campbell, F. A. (1981). Educational intervention for children at risk for mild retardation: A longitudinal analysis. In P. Mittler (Ed.), *Frontiers of knowledge in mental retardation* (Vol. 1). Baltimore: University Park Press.

Rankin, K. (1985a). Hatch: Pay teens less; Senator seeks support for youth wage. *Nation's Restaurant News, 19,* 2.

Rankin, K. (1985b). Subminimum "youth opportunity wage" draws mixed reaction from industry. *Nation's Restaurant News, 19,* 10.

Ratterman, D. (1986). Judicial determination of reasonable efforts. *Children Today, 15,* 28.

Reichelt, P., & Werley, H. (1975). Contraception, abortion, and venereal disease—teenagers' knowledge and the effect of education. *Family Planning Perspectives, 7,* 83–88.

Redmore, C. D., & Loevinger, J. (1979). Ego development in adolescence: Longitudinal studies. *Journal of Youth and Adolescence, 8,* 1–20.

Reiss, I. (1960). *Premarital sex standards in America.* Glencoe, IL: Free Press.

Reiss, I. (1967). *The social context of sexual permissiveness.* New York: Holt, Rinehart & Winston.

Reiss, I. (1976). *Family Systems in America* (2nd ed.). Hinsdale, IL: Dryden Press.

Rickel, A. U. (1986). Prescriptions for a new generation: Early life interventions. *American Journal of Community Psychology, 14,* 1–15.

Rickel, A. U. (1982). Perceptions of adjustment problems in preschool children by teachers and paraprofessional aides. *Journal of Community Psychology, 10,* 29–35.

Rickel, A. U. (1979). *Preschool mental health project: Training manual.* Detroit: State of Michigan, Department of Mental Health.

Rickel, A. U., & Allen L. (1987). *Preventing maladjustment from infancy through adolescence.* Beverly Hills: Sage.

Rickel, A. U., & Biasatti, L. L. (1982). Modification of the Block Child Rearing Practices Report. *Journal of Clinical Psychology, 38,* 129–134.

Rickel, A. U., & Dudley G. (1983). A parent training program in a preschool mental health project. In R. Rosenbaum (Ed.), *Varieties of short term therapy groups: A handbook for mental health professionals.* New York: McGraw-Hill.

Rickel, A. U., Dudley, G., & Berman, S. (1980). An evaluation of parent training. *Evaluation Review, 4,* 389–403.

Rickel, A. U., Gerrard, M., & Iscoe, I. (Eds.). (1984). *Social and psychological problems of women: Prevention and crisis intervention.* Washington, DC: Hemisphere.

Rickel, A. U., & Lampi, L. A. (1981). A two-year follow-up study of a preventive mental health program for preschoolers. *Journal of Abnormal Child Psychology, 9*, 455–464.

Rickel, A. U., & Langner, T. S. (1985). Short- and long-term effects of marital disruption on children. *American Journal of Community Psychology, 13*, 599–611.

Rickel, A. U., Montgomery, E., Thomas, E., Butler, C., Meade, J., & Rowland, L. (1988). *Teenage pregnancy and parenting: Findings from the Detroit Teen Parenting Project.* Paper presented at the American Psychological Association Annual Convention, Atlanta.

Rickel, A. U., & Smith, R. L. (1979). Maladapting preschool children: Identification, diagnosis, and remediation. *American Journal of Community Psychology, 7*, 197–208.

Rickel, A. U., Smith, R. L., & Sharp, K. C. (1979). Description and evaluation of a preventive mental health program for preschoolers. *Journal of Abnormal Child Psychology, 7*, 101–112.

Rickel, A. U., Williams, D. L., & Loigman, G. A. (1988). Predictors of maternal child rearing practices: Implications for intervention. *Journal of Community Psychology, 16*, 32–40.

Rieder, K. (1978). Parents: The unrecognized victims of child abuse. *Military Medicine, 143*(11), 758–762.

Rivera-Casale, C., Klerman, L. V., & Manela, R. (1984). The relevance of child-support enforcement to school-age parents. *Child Welfare, 63*(6), 521–532.

Robert, M. C., & Maddux, J. E. (1982). A psychosocial conceptualization of nonorganic failure to thrive. *Journal of Clinical Child Psychology, 11*, 216–226.

Roberts, M. C., & Peterson, L. (Eds.). (1984). *Prevention of problems in childhood.* New York: John Wiley.

Roberts, R. W. (1966). *The unwed mother.* New York: Harper.

Robertson, E. G. (1981). Adolescence, physiological maturity, and obstetric outcome. In K. Scott, T. Field, & E. Robertson (Eds.), *Teenage parents and their offspring.* New York: Grune & Stratton.

Robinson, I., King, K., & Balsivick, J. (1972). The premarital sexual revolution among college females. *Family Coordinator, 21*, 189–194.

Robinson, I., & Jedlicka, D. (1982). Change in sexual attitudes and behavior of college students from 1967–1980: A research note. *Journal of Marriage and the Family, 44*, 237–240.

Rogel, M., Zuehlke, M., Petersen, A., Tobin-Richards, M., & Shelton, M. (1980). Contraceptive behavior in adolescence: A decision making perspective. *Journal of Youth and Adolescence, 9*, 491–506.

Rogel, M. J., Fleming, J. P., & Zuehlke, M. E. (1981). *Responses to menarche as indicators of sexual attitudes and behaviors.* Paper presented at the annual meeting of the American Psychological Association, Los Angeles.

Rogel, M. J., & Zuehlke, M. E. (1982). Adolescent contraceptive behavior: Influences and implications. In I. R. Stuart and C. F. Wells (Eds.), *Pregnancy in adolescence.* New York: Van Nostrand Reinhold.

Roosa, M. W. (1984). Short-term effects of teenage parenting programs on knowledge and attitudes. *Adolescence, 19*(75), 659–666.

Rosen, B. (1978). Self-concept disturbance among mothers who abuse their children. *Psychology Reports, 43*(1), 323–326.

Rosen, R., Martindale, L., & Grisdela, M. (1976, March). *Pregnancy study report.* Unpublished manuscript. Wayne State University, Detroit.

Rosenberg, M., & Reppucci, N. D. (1983). Abusive mothers: Perceptions of their own and their child's behavior. *Journal of Consulting and Clinical Psychology, 51*(5), 674–682.

Ross, H., & Sawhill, I. (1975). *Time of transition: The growth of families headed by women.* Washington, DC: The Urban Institute.

Rothenberg, P. B. (1978). *Mother-child communication about sex and birth control.* Paper presented at a meeting of the Population Association of America, Atlanta.

Rubin, L. (1976). *Worlds of pain.* New York: Basic Books.

Ruffin, D. (1986). Walking an economic tightrope; an unforeseen downturn in the U. S. economy threatens employment and earning power for black Americans. And the jury is still out on what the future holds for high-tech industries. *Black Enterprise, 16,* 50.

Ruffin, D. C. (1984). The price of youth labor. *Black Enterprise, 15,* 18.

Sacker, I., & Neuhoff, S. D. (1982). Medical and psychosocial risk factors in the pregnant adolescent. In I. R. Stuart & C. F. Wells (Eds.), *Pregnancy in adolescence* (pp. 107–139). New York: Van Nostrand Reinhold.

Sameroff, A. J., & Chandler, M. J. (1975). Reproductive risk and the continuum of caretaking causality. In F. D. Horowitz, M. Heterington, S. Scarr-Salapatek, & G. Siegel (Eds.), *Review of child development research* (Vol. 4). Chicago: University of Chicago Press.

Sameroff, A. J., Seifer, R., Zax, M., & Barocas, R. (1987). *Schizophrenia Bulletin, 13*(3), 383–394.

Sauber, M., & Corrigan, E. (1970). *The six-year experience of unwed mothers as parents.* New York: Community Council of Greater New York.

Scales, P., & Beckstein, D. (1982). From macho to mutuality: Helping young men make effective decisions about sex, contraception, and pregnancy. In I. Stuart & C. Wells (Eds.), *Pregnancy in adolescence* (pp. 264–289). New York: Van Nostrand Reinhold.

Schenkel, S., & Marcia, J. (1972). Attitudes toward premarital intercourse in determining ego identity status in college women. *Journal of Personality, 3,* 472–482.

Schinke, S. P. (1982). School-based model for preventing teenage pregnancy. *Social Work in Education, 4,* 34–42.

Schmidt, A. V. (1985). Teenage mothers; School-based child care puts diploma in reach. *Children Today, 14,* 16.

Segal, S. M., & Ducette, J. (1973). Locus of control and pre-marital high-school pregnancy. *Psychological Reports, 33*(3), 887–890.

Shah, F., Zelnick, M., & Kantner, J. (1975). Unprotected intercourse among unwed teenagers. *Family Planning Perspectives, 7,* 39.

Sharples, S. (1986). Cue! for training young people. *Retail & Distribution, 14,* 42.

Sheets, K. (1986, July 7). Teen jobs go begging this summer. *U. S. News & World Report,* 59.

Sigman, M., & Parmelee, A. H. (1979). Longitudinal evaluation of the preterm infant. In T. M. Field, A. M. Sostek, S. Goldberg, & H. H. Shuman (Eds.), *Infants born at risk*. New York: Spectrum.

Simpkins, L. (1984). Consequences of teenage pregnancy and motherhood. *Adolescence, 19*(73), 39–51.

Simmons, R. G., Rosenberg, F., & Rosenberg, M. (1973). Disturbance in the self image at adolescence. *American Sociological Review, 38,* 553–568.

Simmons, R. G., Blyth, D. A., VanCleave, E. F., & Bush, D. M. (1979). Entry into early adolescence: The impact of school structure, puberty, and early dating on self-esteem. *American Sociological Review, 44,* 948–967.

Simmons, R. G., Blyth, D. A., Carlton-Ford, S., & Bulcroft, R. (1982). *The adjustment of early adolescents to school and pubertal transitions*. Paper presented at a meeting of the Life Span Development Committee of the Social Science Research Council, Tucson.

Singh, B. (1980). Trends in attitudes toward premarital sexual relationships. *Journal of Marriage and the Family, 42,* 387–394.

Siqueland, E. R. (1973). Biological and experiential determinants of exploration in infancy. In L. J. Stone, J. T. Smith, & L. B. Murphy (Eds.), *The competent infant*. New York: Basic Books.

Smith, P. B., & Mumford, D. M. (Eds.) (1980). *Adolescent pregnancy: Prespective of the health professional*. Boston: G. K. Hale.

Spanier, G. (1975). Sexualization and premarital sexual behaviors. *Family Coordinator, 24,* 33–41.

Sorensen, R. (1973). *Adolescent sexuality in contemporary America*. New York: World Publishing.

Staples, R. (1973). *The black woman in America: Sex, marriage and the family*. Chicago: Nelson-Hall.

Stark, E. (1986, October). Young, innocent and pregnant. *Psychology Today*, pp. 28–35.

Steinlauf, B. (1979). Problem-solving skills, locus of control, and the contraceptive effectiveness of young women. *Child Development, 50,* 268–271.

Stevens, J. S. (1988). Social support, locus of control, and parenting in three low income groups of mothers: Black teenagers, black adults, and white adults. *Child Development, 59,* 635–642.

Sudia, C. (1986). Preventing out-of-home placement of children: The first step to permanency planning. *Children Today, 15,* 4.

Tamashiro, R. T. (1979). Adolescents' concept of marriage: A structural-developmental analysis. *Journal of Youth and Adolescence, 8*(4), 643–652.

Tanner, J. M. (1970). Physical development. In P. H. Mussen (Ed.), *Carmichael's manual of child psychology* (Vol. I) (pp. 77–156). New York: Wiley.

Tauer, K. M. (1983). Promoting effective decision-making in sexually active adolescents. *Nursing Clinics of North America, 18,* 275–292.

Terman, L. (1938). *Psychological factors in marital happiness*. New York: McGraw-Hill.

Thomas, E. A. (1988). *MMPI personality subtypes and parenting styles among teenage mothers*. Unpublished master's thesis, Wayne State University, Detroit.

Tietze, C. (1975). Contraceptive practice in the context of a nonrestrictive abortion law: Age-specific pregnancy rates in New York City, 1971–1973. *Family Planning Perspectives, 7*, 197–202.

Tiggaman, M., & Winsfield, A. H. (1984). The effects of unemployment on the mood, self-esteem, locus of control, and depressive affect of school-leavers. *Journal of Occupational Psychology, 57*, 33.

Tobin-Richards, H. M., Boxer, A. M., & Petersen, A. C. (1983). The psychological significance of pubertal change: Sex differences in perceptions of self during early adolescence. In J. Brooks-Gunn & A. C. Petersen (Eds.), *Girls at puberty: Biological and psychosocial perspectives*. New York: Plenum Press.

Toder, N. L., & Marcia, J. E. (1973). Ego identity status and response to conformity pressure in college women. *Journal of Personality and Social Psychology, 26*, 287–294.

Torres, A., Forrest, J. D., & Eisman, S. (1981). Family planning services in the United States, 1978–1979. *Family Planning Perspectives, 13*, 132–141.

Treiman, R. (1986). *Infant attachment in children of teen mothers*. Unpublished manuscript, Merrill-Palmer Institute, Detroit.

Turkel, S. B., & Abramson, T. (1986). Peer tutoring and mentoring as a drop-out prevention strategy. *Clearing House, 60*, 68.

Udry, J. (1983). *Socialization of adolescent sexual behavior*. Chapel Hill: Carolina Population Center, University of North Carolina.

Udry, J., Bauman, K., & Morris, N. (1975). Changes in premarital coital experience of recent decades of birth cohorts of urban America. *Journal of Marriage and the Family, 37*, 783–787.

U. S. Bureau of the Census. (1982). *Characteristics of the population below the poverty level: 1980* (Current Population Reports, Series P-60, No. 133). Washington, DC: U. S. Government Printing Office.

Vener, A., & Stewart, C. (1974). Adolescent sexual behavior in middle America revisited: 1970–1973. *Journal of Marriage and the Family, 36*, 728–735.

Vincent, C. (1961). *Unmarried mothers*. London: Free Press.

Vukelich, C., & Kliman, D. (1985). Mature and teenage mothers' infant growth expectations and use of child development information sources. *Family Relations, 34*, 189–196.

Waddill, D. (1984). Teens and adoption: A pregnancy resolution alternative? *Children Today, 13*, 24.

Wäde, R. (1977). *For men about abortion*. Boulder, CO: Author.

Webster-Stratton, C. (1987). Modifications of mothers' behaviors and attitudes through a video modeling group discussion program. *Behavior Therapy, 12*(5), 634–642.

Weigle, J. (1976, January/February). Teaching child development to teenage mothers. *Illinois Teacher*, 157–159.

Werner, E. E., Bierman, J. M., & French, F. E. (1971). *The children of Kauai*. Honolulu: University Press of Hawaii.

Werner, E. E., & Smith, R. S. (1977). *Kauai's children come of age*. Honolulu: University Press of Hawaii.

Westoff, C. F., Calot, G., & Foster, A. D. (1983). Teenage fertility in developed nations: 1971–1980. *Family Planning Perspectives, 15*, 105–110.

Widmayer, S., & Field T. (1980). Effects of Brazelton demonstrations on early interactions of preterm infants and their mothers. *Infant Behavior and Development, 3*, 79–89.

Williams, D. R. (1984). Young discouraged workers: Racial differences explored. *Monthly Labor Review, 107*, 36.

Wilkinson, C. B., & O'Connor, W. A. (1977). Growing up male in a black single-parent family. *Psychiatric Annals, 7*(7), 50–59.

Yalom, I. D., Lunde, D. T., Moos, R. H., & Hamburg, D. (1968). "Post partum blues" syndrome. *Archives of General Psychiatry, 18*, 16–27.

Yankelovich, D. (1974). *The new morality: A profile of American youth in the 1970's*. New York: McGraw-Hill.

Yankelovich, Skelly, & White, Inc. (1979). *The General Mills American Family Report, 1978–1979: Family health in an era of stress*. Minneapolis: General Mills.

Yin, R. K. (1984). *Case study research: Design and methods*. Beverly Hills: Sage.

Zabin, L. S., & Clark, S. D. (1981). Why they delay: A study of teenage planning clinic patients. *Family Planning Perspectives, 13*, 205–217.

Zabin, L. S., Hardy, J. B., Streett, R., & King, T. M. (1984). A school-, hospital- and university-based pregnancy prevention program. *The Journal of Reproductive Medicine, 29*, 421–426.

Zabin, L. S., Hirsch, M. B., Smith, E. A., & Hardy, J. B. (1984). Adolescent sexual attitudes and behavior: Are they consistent? *Family Planning Perspectives, 16*, 181–185.

Zabin, L. S., Hirsch, M. B., Smith, E. A., Streett, R., & Hardy, J. B. (1986a). Adolescent pregnancy-prevention program: A model for research and evaluation. *Journal of Adolescent Health Care, 7*, 77–87.

Zabin, L. S., Hirsch, M. B., Smith, E. A., Streett, R., & Hardy, J. B. (1986b). Evaluation of a pregnancy prevention program for urban teenagers. *Family Planning Perspectives, 18*, 119–126.

Zelnik, M., & Kantner, J. F. (1977). Sexual and contraceptive experience of young unmarried women in the United States, 1976 and 1971. *Family Planning Perspectives, 9*, 55–71.

Zelnik, M., & Kantner, J. F. (1978). Contraceptive patterns and premarital pregnancy among women aged 15–19 in 1976. *Family Planning Perspectives, 10*, 135–142.

Zelnik, M., & Kantner, J. (1979). Sex education and knowledge of pregnancy risk among U. S. teenage women. *Family Planning Perspectives, 11*, 355–357.

Zelnik, M., & Kantner, J. (1980). Sexuality, contraception and pregnancy among young unwed females in the United States. In *Research Reports* (Vol. I). Commission on Population Growth and the American Future. Washington, DC: U. S. Government Printing Office.

Zelnik, M., & Kantner, J. F. (1980). Sexual activity, contraceptive use and pregnancy among metropolitan area teenagers: 1971–1979. *Family Planning Perspectives, 12*, 230–237.

Zelnik, M., Kantner, J., & Ford, K. (1981). *Sex and pregnancy in adolescence.* Beverly Hills: Sage.

Zelnik, M., Kantner, J., & Ford, K. (1982). *Adolescent pathways to pregnancy.* Beverly Hills: Sage.

Zelnik, M., & Kim, Y. J. (1982). Sex education and its association with teenage sexual activity, pregnancy and contraceptive use. *Family Planning Perspectives, 14,* 117–126.

Ziglor, E., & Rubin, N. (1985). Why child abuse occurs: Stress, isolation, or ignorance of the developmental patterns of children—not craziness—make for abuse. *Parents, 6,* 102.

Zonger, C. E. (1977). The self concept of pregnant adolescent girls. *Adolescence, 12*(48), 477–488.

Zuravin, S. (1988). Child maltreatment and teenage first births: A relationship mediated by chronic sociodemographic stress? *American Journal of Orthopsychiatry, 58,* 91.

Appendix

Dear Respondent: Thank you in advance for your cooperation. We sincerely appreciate the time and effort you are contributing to this valuable project.

CONSENT FORM

I consent to be interviewed by the Parenting Project. I understand that the purpose of this project is to study how the social environment (home, friends, school, community services) influences behavior. This study could make a major contribution to the fields of education, health, family life, human development, and urban planning. There are no apparent risks or discomforts from participating in it.

I understand that I may refuse to answer any questions and that I may discontinue my participation at any time. I further understand that every reply will be treated in the strictest confidence and numerical codes will be used instead of names. The replies I give will be seen only by the research staff.

If I have any questions about the research, either now or in the future, I should feel free to contact the office of Dr. Annette U. Rickel at 577-2859.

_____   _____
        Date   Signature of Respondent

QUESTIONNAIRE

_____   Case Number
Respondent's Name   _____

Your present address is _____
                        Street Address

_____
City   State   Zip

_____
Telephone (area code and number)

1.   What type of housing is that?   House/mobile home   1
                                           Apartment   2
                                           Rooming house   3
                                           School dormitory, etc.   4
                                           Flat   5

2.   Could you tell me who you live with and what their relationship is to you? I'd also
      like to know the age of each person in your household.

      (List R's household composition. If R is married, note spouse; if R has children in
      the household, list them and any other people living there. If R is living with a
      roommate or relative, list that person or persons.)

People in R's Household

Name	Age	Sex M F	(Enter 2 digits from code list.*) Relationship to R:
a. _____		1 2	_____
b. _____		1 2	_____
c. _____		1 2	_____
d. _____		1 2	_____
e. _____		1 2	_____
f. _____		1 2	_____
g. _____		1 2	_____
h. _____		1 2	_____
i. _____		1 2	_____

*Relationship Codes

Lover**	31	Mother-in-law	13	Roomer	25
Husband	01	Father-in-law	14	Friend, casual	26
Wife	02	Brother	15	Grandmother	27
Natural daughter	03	Sister	16	Grandfather	28
Natural son	04	Brother-in-law	17	Grandmother-in-law	29
Stepdaughter	05	Sister-in-law	18	Grandfather-in-law	30
Stepson	06	Aunt	19	Stepbrother	32
Adopted daughter	07	Uncle	20	Stepsister	33
Adopted son	08	Aunt-in-law	21	Half brother	34
Foster daughter	09	Uncle-in-law	22	Half sister	35
Foster son	10	Cousin	23	Stepfather	36
Mother	11	Cousin-in-law	24	Stepmother	37
Father	12				

(**Close emotional relationship)

3. That makes a total of _____ people in your household.
   (Enter number. Include R in the total count.)

4. How long have you lived at this address? a. _____

                                        (years)

                                     b. _____

                                        (months)

5. Now I'd like to inquire about your current marital status. Are you now

Single?	1
Married?	2
Divorced?	3
Separated?	4
Abandoned?	5
Widowed?	6
Common law, legal?	7

6a. Do you have children who are not living with you?
   (If *yes* answer 6b.)

No	1
Yes, permanent separation (e.g., adoption)	2
Yes, temporary separation or divorce	3

6b.   Name   Age   Sex
                                                                                M   F
    a. _____   1   2
    _____
    b. _____   1   2
    _____

7. How many times have you been pregnant?   _____

8. How did pregnancy end?

	a. First time	b. Second time	c. Third time
Baby born, kept by R _____	1	1	1
Baby born, adopted _____	2	2	2
Baby born, cared for by parents or other family _____	3	3	3
Aborted, spontaneous _____	4	4	4
Aborted, legal _____	5	5	5
Aborted, other _____	6	6	6
Baby unborn _____	7	7	7

9. (If R had and kept child ask:) What was your marital status at the time of birth?
    (Probe for "to whom married.")

	a. First time	b. Second time	c. Third time
R married to child's father at time of birth _____	1	1	1
R married to child's father after birth _____	2	2	2
R not married _____	3	3	3
R married not to child's father _____	4	4	4

Now we need an update on your family to complete this section.

	Living	Deceased
10. Could you tell me about your parents? Is your mother still living?	1	2
11. And your father?	1	2

12. What about your siblings?
    (Specify each sibling's name and code.)

	Living	Deceased
a. _____	1	2
b. _____	1	2
c. _____	1	2
d. _____	1	2
e. _____	1	2

13. Are your parents living together?

Married and living together	1
Separated	2
Divorced	3
Never married	4
Mother deceased	5
Father deceased	6

(Ask only if R is from a broken family.)

	Yes	No
14. Did either of your parents remarry in the past 10 years? What about your mother?	1	2
15. What about your father?	1	2

I'd like to ask you some questions about what you are doing now in terms of work or school.

16. Are you working now? (If on paid vacation or paid sick leave from job, code for working.)

Yes	1
No	2

17. What kind of work do you do now?

Professional/technical	1
Manager, administrator, clerical, or sales	2
Craftsman, foreman	3
Service worker, housekeeper, farmer	4
Unskilled laborer	5
Not in work force	6

18. Is your present job full- or part-time?

Full-time	1
Part-time	2

(*Note:* If part-time, ask:)

19. How many hours per week do you work on average?
(Code number) _____

20. How do you support yourself?

Unemployment insurance	1
(*Note:* Check ADC if ADC and parents. Check Social Security if parents and Social Security.) Ward of court/residential home aid/ student on educational assistance	2
Disability benefits/Social Security	3
Housewife or spouse supports	4
Parents/self are supporting	5
ADC/Medicaid/WIC	6

21. Are you now attending a school of any type?

Yes	1
No	2

Next we would like to ask you some questions about your schooling.

(If yes, ask 22–26.)

22. What type of school is it?

(*Note*: Alternative school = high school equivalency.)

High school	1
High school equivalency	2
Trade	3
College	4
Adult education courses	5

23. Do you go to school full- or part-time?

Full-time	1
Part-time	2

24. Have you been able to keep up with your classwork in the last 3 months? Would you say you keep up

Very well?	5
Well?	4
Average?	3
Poorly?	2
Not at all?	1

25. How many days in the last 3 months were you absent from school because you just didn't feel like going? Would you say

Seven or more times?	1
Five or six times?	2
Three or four times?	3
One or two times?	4
Zero times?	5

26. What have your grades averaged in the current or previous semester—that is, what was your grade point average?

a. _____
(Grade point average)

b. _____
(On a scale of)

Here are some questions about religion.

27. To what religious faith do you now belong? (If any reply is Protestant, get and circle specific denomination. If Jewish, ask "Orthodox, Conservative, or Reform?")

Catholic	1	Eastern/Greek/ Russian Orthodox	17
Jewish Orthodox	2	Pentecostal	18
Jewish Conservative	3	Jehovah Witness	19
Jewish Reform	4	Church of God in Christ	20
Jewish, other	5	Seventh Day Adventist	21
Episcopal	6	Christian Scientist	22
Presbyterian	7	Mormon	23
Unitarian	11	Christian, nondenominational	24
Congregational	12	Muhammadan	25
Methodist	13	Hindu	26
Lutheran	14	Other	27
Baptist	15	None	28
Other Protestant	16		

28. How often do you attend religious services?

Daily	Once a week	Few times a month	Once a month	Few times a year	Once a year	Less than once a year	Never
1	2	3	4	5	6	7	11

To what extent do you agree or disagree with the following statements of religious belief?

	Agree strongly	Agree	Disagree	Disagree strongly
29. Without belief in God life is meaningless. Do you agree strongly, agree, disagree, or disagree strongly?	1	2	3	4
30. When in doubt, it's best to stop and ask God what to do. Do you agree strongly, agree, disagree, or disagree strongly?	1	2	3	4

31. Belief in God helps make you
a stronger and better person.
Do you agree strongly, agree,
disagree, or disagree
strongly?   1   2   3   4

32. With what racial and ethnic grouping do you identify most strongly?

White	1	Italian
	2	Eastern European
	3	Irish
	4	English
	5	Other European
	6	South American/Central American
	7	Islander (including Puerto Rico and Cuba)
	8	Spanish
	11	Other (specify) _____
Black	12	United States
	13	West Indies (Jamaica, Haiti, etc.)
	14	African
Asian	16	Chinese
	17	Japanese
	18	Indian

33. Have you had any illnesses that required hospitalization in the past 10 years?

Yes   1

No   2

(If yes, ask:)
34. What?   When?

Chronic illness	2	_____
Viral problems	3	_____
Accident	4	_____
Gynecological	5	_____
Sexually transmitted disease	6	_____
Blood related	7	_____
Surgery	8	_____

35. Do you have regular physical examinations?

Yes	1
No	2

36. When was your last examination?
a. _____ (Month)   b. _____ (Year)
   (Enter approximate month and year.)

37. Do you have regular dental examinations?

Yes	1
No	2

38. When was your last examination?
a. _____ (Month)   b. _____ (Year)
   (Enter approximate month and year.)

39. During your last pregnancy how often did you go for checkups?

Seven or more times	1
Five or six times	2
Three or four times	3
One or two times	4
Zero times	5

40. Did you have any physical problems during your pregnancy?

No	1
Yes	
Chronic illness	3
Viral	4
Accident	5
Gynecological	6
Sexual transmitted disease	7
Blood related	8
Surgery	9

41. Have you used any of the following during your pregnancy? Enter in one box
   only.

	No	No. of times daily	No. of times weekly	No. of times monthly
Tobacco				
Alcohol				
Illegal drugs				
Prescribed medication (specify)				
Over-the-counter medication (specify)				

42. Were there complications with the baby's birth?

No	1
Yes	
Genetic	3
Prenatal	4
Perinatal	5

43. What was the sex, size, and Apgar score of the baby?

	M	F	Weight	Height	Apgar
a. Baby	1	2			
b. Twin	1	2			
c. Triplet	1	2			

44. Was the baby full term (9 months)?

a. Yes	1
b. No	2
Specify months/weeks premature	

_____

45. Did the baby have any physical abnormalities?

a. No	1
b. Yes	
Genetic	3
Prenatal	4
Perinatal	5

46. Are you breastfeeding your baby?

a. No	1
b. Yes	2

47. How satisfied have you been with the kind of mother you are—would you say

Very satisfied	4
Somewhat satisfied	3
Somewhat dissatisfied	2
Very dissatisfied	1
Don't know	0

48. How satisfied have you been as a parent with how well you understand your baby's needs?

Very satisfied	4
Somewhat satisfied	3
Somewhat dissatisfied	2
Very dissatisfied	1
Don't know	0

49. How satisfied have you been with how you get along with your baby?

Very satisfied	4
Somewhat satisfied	3
Somewhat dissatisfied	2
Very dissatisfied	1
Don't know	0

50. How satisfied have you been as a mother with the time spent with your baby?

Very satisfied	4
Somewhat satisfied	3
Somewhat dissatisfied	2
Very dissatisfied	1
Don't know	0

51. When you compare yourself to other mothers with babies your child's age, how well do you think you have done? Would you say

Far above average	4
Above average	3
Average	2
Somewhat below average	1
Far below average	0

52. What was your relationship with the baby's father when you got pregnant?

Committed relationship	4
Good friends	3
Casual friends	2
Barely knew	1

53. Do you use birth control?

Pill	1	Sponge	5
Condom	2	Spermicide	6
Diaphragm	3	Other	7
IUD	4	None	8

54. How did you feel when you learned that you were pregnant?

Happy	1	Disgusted	5
Scared	2	Confused/mixed feelings	6
Unhappy/disappointed	3	Denial	7
Shocked	4		

55. How did the baby's father feel?

Happy	1	Disgusted	5
Scared	2	Confused/mixed feelings	6
Unhappy/disappointed	3	Denial	7
Shocked	4	Unaware	8

AVERAGE BABY[*]

Although this is your first baby, you probably have some idea of what most little babies are like. Please check the blank you think best describes the *average* baby.

How much crying do you think the average baby does?

A great deal	A good bit	Moderate amount	Very little	None

How much trouble do you think the average baby has in feeding?

A great deal	A good bit	Moderate amount	Very little	None

How much spitting up or vomiting do you think the average baby does?

A great deal	A good bit	Moderate amount	Very little	None

[*] From E. R. Broussard & M. S. Hartner, Further considerations regarding maternal perceptions of the first born. In J. Hellmuth (Ed.), *Exceptional infant, Vol. 2: Studies in abnormalities.* New York: Brunner Mazel. Copyright 1964 by Elsie R. Broussard, MD. Reprinted with permission from Elsie R. Broussard. Readers should contact Elsie R. Broussard for permission to use the inventories.

How much difficulty do you think the average baby has with sleeping?

| _____ | _____ | _____ | _____ | _____ |
| A great deal | A good bit | Moderate amount | Very little | None |

How much difficulty does the average baby have with bowel movements?

| _____ | _____ | _____ | _____ | _____ |
| A great deal | A good bit | Moderate amount | Very little | None |

How much trouble do you think the average baby has in settling down to a predictable pattern of eating and sleeping?

| _____ | _____ | _____ | _____ | _____ |
| A great deal | A good bit | Moderate amount | Very little | None |

YOUR BABY[*]

You have had a chance to live with your baby for a while[**] now. Please check the blank you think best describes *your* baby.

How much crying has your baby done?

| _____ | _____ | _____ | _____ | _____ |
| A great deal | A good bit | Moderate amount | Very little | None |

How much trouble has your baby had with feeding?

| _____ | _____ | _____ | _____ | _____ |
| A great deal | A good bit | Moderate amount | Very little | None |

How much spitting up or vomiting has your baby done?

| _____ | _____ | _____ | _____ | _____ |
| A great deal | A good bit | Moderate amount | Very little | None |

How much difficulty has your baby had in sleeping?

| _____ | _____ | _____ | _____ | _____ |
| A great deal | A good bit | Moderate amount | Very little | None |

[*] From E. R. Broussard & M. S. Hartner, Further consideration regarding maternal perceptions of the first born. In J. Hellmuth (Ed.), *Exceptional Infant, Vol. 2: Studies in abnormalities*. New York: Brunner Mazel. Copyright 1964 by Elsie R. Broussard, MD. Reprinted with permission from Elsie R. Broussard. Readers should contact Elsie R. Broussard for permission to use the inventories.

[**]Modified from the original which reads *a month*.

How much difficulty has your baby had with bowel movements?

A great deal	A good bit	Moderate amount	Very little	None

How much trouble has your baby had in settling down to a predictable pattern of eating and sleeping?

A great deal	A good bit	Moderate amount	Very little	None

Listed below are some of the things that have sometimes bothered other parents in caring for their babies. We would like to know if you are bothered by any of these. Please place a check mark in the blank that best describes how much you are bothered by your baby's behavior in regard to these.

Crying

A great deal	Somewhat	Very little	None

Spitting up or vomiting

A great deal	Somewhat	Very little	None

Sleeping

A great deal	Somewhat	Very little	None

Feeding

A great deal	Somewhat	Very little	None

Elimination

A great deal	Somewhat	Very little	None

Lack of predictable schedule

A great deal	Somewhat	Very little	None

*Unresponsive

A great deal	Somewhat	Very little	None

Demanding

A great deal	Somewhat	Very little	None

Irritable

A great deal	Somewhat	Very little	None

Excessively active

A great deal	Somewhat	Very little	None

*Last four items replaced the category *other.*

MOTHER'S OPINION MEASURE (MOM)

1. It has been a long day and you still have to do the grocery shopping with your baby along. You want to go in and get it done as quickly and easily as possible. Your baby starts fussing as soon as you go into the grocery store. In the beginning he/she is just complaining and trying to get out of the cart. As you go down the aisles he/she gets louder and louder. Your baby starts chewing on packages and throwing them out of the cart. Before you can finish your shopping he/she is throwing an all-out temper tantrum. Everyone is turning to look at you. How would you handle the problem?

2. You have friends coming over in an hour, and it is time for your baby to go to bed. You have gone through the normal bedtime ritual, but your baby refuses to go to bed. At first your baby acts like it is a game and wants you to chase him/her. After this your baby starts screaming and crying about going to bed. You put your baby into bed anyway and he/she continues to scream and cry. What would you do?

3. You are going to a party. You are really looking forward to it because it's been a long time since you've gotten together with your friends or been anywhere without your baby. You know you're going to have a great time. You've bought yourself something new to wear and are excited about this party. Just as you are about to leave the baby gets into a chocolate bar you have in your purse. You go to get him/her away from it, and the baby grabs you and gets chocolate all over your clothes. What would you do?

4. Your baby is playing on the floor with your friend's baby. They seemed to be playing nicely but all of a sudden you hear crying. You run out of the bathroom and see that they are both crying and grabbing for the same Big Bird doll. What would you do?

5. Your toddler is a great climber. Every time he/she gets the chance he/she climbs up onto the dining room table. More than anything else you are scared that he/she will fall off of it and hurt him/herself, but of course you also want your toddler to learn that the table is not something to play on. You feel like you've said *no* a hundred times. What could you do that might work?

6. It seems as though everyone is into physical fitness today, and you realize that even a baby may need help to develop physically. Since it is important for your baby's muscles to develop properly, can you list some toys and activities that could help your baby develop his/her muscles?

7. Any parent can be overwhelmed when they walk into a store like Toys R' Us or Children's Palace. There is such a choice and variety of toys for children, and there is no way anybody could possibly buy them all. However, this does give parents the feeling that maybe their child is missing out on something. List some toys or games that can easily be made.

8. Mary loves her baby very much, but rarely talks to him/her. Since the baby doesn't speak yet she doesn't think the baby can understand what she's saying. Mary has bought storybooks to read to the baby but is waiting for the time when she thinks he/she can understand and enjoy them. How do you feel about this?

9. Describe a typical day in your baby's life.

Activities

Morning	
Afternoon	
Evening	
Bedtime	
Night	

10. Plan a day's meals and snacks for a 1-year-old.

PERCEIVED SOCIAL SUPPORT NETWORK INVENTORY*

The support we receive from family, friends, professional helpgivers, and others during times of stress seems to play an important role in determining our reaction to that stress. The interaction that we have with supportive individuals appears to help us feel better faster after, for example, flunking an exam, having difficulties with the baby, or experiencing a conflict with someone. This questionnaire attempts to gather information about your perceptions and experiences with your support network in response to stressful events that have occurred in your life.

Support Network

Write the first name and last initial of all the people you would go to if you needed support or help during a stressful time in your life. Check the appropriate column that describes your relationship with each person. You do not have to fill out this list in any order. You do not have to use all the spaces available.

		1	2	3	4	5	6	7
	First name, last initial	Spouse or partner	Family member	Friend	Co-worker	Professional helpgiver	Religious leader	Self-help group
1								
2								
3								
4								
5								
6								
7								

Helping Behaviors

Support from people during stressful events can be broken down into six categories of helping behaviors:

* From E. Oritt, S. Paul, & J. Behrmann, The perceived support network inventory. *American Journal of Community Psychology, 13*(5), 565–582. Copyright 1985. Reprinted with permission.

1. *Emotional support*—someone listening to your private thoughts and feelings regarding a stressful event and/or giving you physical affection.

2. *Material aid support*—someone lending you money or the use of some valuable object such as a car or an appliance during a stressful event.

3. *Advice and information*—someone suggesting what to do or where to get needed information during a stressful event.

4. *Physical assistance*—someone helping with jobs around the house, errands, favors you might need during a stressful event.

5. *Social participation*—someone offering you the opportunity to engage in pleasant social activities during a stressful event.

6. *Parenting support*—someone helping with feeding, diapering, clothing, soothing, or entertaining your baby.

Support Network Information

On the following pages are questions about the people whose names you wrote down on the *Support Network* list. Please write the first name and last initial of the *first person* you listed and answer the questions about him/her. Then write the first name and last initial of the *second person* you listed and answer the questions about him/her. Go through your entire *Support Network* list. Each set of questions for each person takes less than a minute to answer, so the following pages will not take you long.

First name, last initial _____ Code 1–7

Rate the extent to which you agree with the following statements by circling the appropriate numbers.

	Almost never	Sometimes	Usually	Almost always			
During times of stress:							
I seek this person out for support or help	1	2	3	4	5	6	7
This person provides me with support or help when I ask	1	2	3	4	5	6	7
I am satisfied with this person's support or help	1	2	3	4	5	6	7

Place a check next to the categories of support you might expect to receive from this person during times of stress:

_____ a. Emotional support   _____ d. Physical assistance
_____ b. Material aid support   _____ e. Social participation
_____ c. Advice and information   _____ f. Parenting support

This person receives support from me during times of stress for him/her.

1	2	3	4	5	6	7
Almost never		Sometimes		Usually		Almost always

Generally speaking, I have serious conflicts with this person.

7	6	5	4	3	2	1
Almost never		Sometimes		Usually		Almost always

This person helps me care for my baby an average of
a. _____ times daily   c. _____ times monthly
b. _____ times weekly   d. _____ no times

RICKEL MODIFIED CHILD REARING PRACTICES REPORT (R-CRPR)[*]

In answering the following questions consider how you treat your child now and will in the future.

1	2	3	4	5	6
Not at all descriptive of me	Slightly	Somewhat	Fairly	Very	Highly descriptive of me

1. I respect my child's opinions and encourage him/her to express them.   1 2 3 4 5 6

2. I don't think that children of different sexes should be allowed to see each other naked.   1 2 3 4 5 6

3. I feel that a child should be given comfort and understanding when he/she is scared or upset.   1 2 3 4 5 6

4. I try to keep my child away from children or families whose ideas or values are different from our own.   1 2 3 4 5 6

5. I believe that a child should be seen and not heard.   1 2 3 4 5 6

6. I express affection by hugging, kissing, and holding my child.   1 2 3 4 5 6

*Adapted from J. Block (1965). _The child rearing practices report._

7. I find some of my greatest satisfaction in my child.   1 2 3 4 5 6

8. I encourage my child to wonder and think about life.   1 2 3 4 5 6

9. I usually take into account my child's preference   1 2 3 4 5 6
    when making plans for the family.

10. I feel that a child should have time to daydream,   1 2 3 4 5 6
    think, and even loaf sometimes.

11. I do not allow my child to say bad things about his/her   1 2 3 4 5 6
    teacher.

12. I teach my child that in one way or another punish-   1 2 3 4 5 6
    ment will find him/her when he is bad.

13. I do not allow my child to get angry with me.   1 2 3 4 5 6

14. I am easygoing and relaxed with my child.   1 2 3 4 5 6

15. I talk it over and reason with my child when he/she   1 2 3 4 5 6
    misbehaves.

16. I trust my child to behave as he/she should, even   1 2 3 4 5 6
    when I am not with him/her.

17. I joke and play with my child.   1 2 3 4 5 6

18. My child and I have warm, intimate moments to-   1 2 3 4 5 6
    gether.

19. I encourage my child to be curious, to explore, and to   1 2 3 4 5 6
    question things.

20. I expect my child to be grateful and appreciate all   1 2 3 4 5 6
    advantages he/she has.

21. I believe in toilet training a child as soon as possible.   1 2 3 4 5 6

22. I believe in praising a child when he/she is good and   1 2 3 4 5 6
    think it gets better results than punishing him/her
    when he/she is bad.

23. I make sure my child knows that I appreciate what he/   1 2 3 4 5 6
    she tries to accomplish.

24. I encourage my child to talk about his/her troubles.   1 2 3 4 5 6

25. I believe children should not have secrets from their parents.   1   2   3   4   5   6

26. I teach my child to keep control of his/her feelings at all times.   1   2   3   4   5   6

27. I dread answering my child's questions about sex.   1   2   3   4   5   6

28. When I am angry with my child, I let him/her know about it.   1   2   3   4   5   6

29. I think a child should be encouraged to do things better than others.   1   2   3   4   5   6

30. I believe that scolding and criticism make a child improve.   1   2   3   4   5   6

31. I believe a child should be aware of how much I sacrifice for him/her.   1   2   3   4   5   6

32. I do not allow my child to question my decisions.   1   2   3   4   5   6

33. I let my child know how ashamed and disappointed I am when he/she misbehaves.   1   2   3   4   5   6

34. I want my child to make a good impression on others.   1   2   3   4   5   6

35. I find it interesting and educational to be with my child for long periods.   1   2   3   4   5   6

36. I instruct my child not to get dirty when he/she is playing.   1   2   3   4   5   6

37. I control my child by warning him/her about the bad things that can happen to him/her.   1   2   3   4   5   6

38. I don't want my child to be looked on as different from others.   1   2   3   4   5   6

39. I prefer my child not try things if there is a chance he/she might fail.   1   2   3   4   5   6

40. I don't think children should be given information on sex.   1   2   3   4   5   6

LIFE EVENTS SCALE[*]

Now I'll ask you about experiences that people have. Some of these things happen to most people at one time or another, while some of these things happen to only a few people. I'll ask you about experiences that you have had in the last year since _____.

                                                                    Month/Year

The first questions are about *schooling*.

1. Since _____ did either of these things happen to you?

        Month/Year

(Circle proper code. For each *yes* circled, do follow-up probe when all life events are completed.)

	Yes	
	R	No

| a. | Started school or a training program after not going to school for a long time | 1 | 9 |
| b. | Graduated from school or training program | 1 | 9 |

Here are some events related to *work*.

2. Since _____ did any of these things happen to you?

        Month/Year

a.	Started work for the first time	1	9
b.	Returned to work after not working for a long time	1	9
c.	Changed jobs for a better one	1	9
d.	Changed jobs for a worse one	1	9
e.	Had trouble with a boss	1	9
f.	Demoted at work	1	9
g.	Found out that was *not* going to be promoted at work	1	9
h.	Promoted	1	9
i.	Had significant or important success in work	1	9

[*] From B. S. Dohwenrend & B. P. Dohwenrend, *Stressful life events: Their nature and effects.* New York: Wiley. Copyright 1974. Reprinted with permission.

j.	Laid off	1	9
k.	Fired	1	9
l.	Started a business or profession	1	9
m.	Expanded business or professional practice	1	9
n.	Suffered a business loss or failure	1	9
o.	Sharply reduced workload	1	9
p.	Retired	1	9
q.	Stopped working, but *not* retired, for an extended period	1	9

Here are some events related to *love and marriage.*

3. Since _____ did any of these things happen to you?
Month/Year

a.	Became engaged	1	9
b.	Engagement broken	1	9
c.	Married	1	9
d.	Started a love affair	1	9
e.	Relations with spouse changed for the worse, without separation or divorce	1	9
f.	Married couple separated	1	9
g.	Divorced	1	9
h.	Relations with spouse changed for the better	1	9
i.	R—Engaged in marital infidelity	1	9
j.	Spouse engaged in infidelity	1	9
k.	Spouse died	1	9
l.	Got togther with spouse again after separation	1	9

Here are some events related to *having children.*

4. Since _____ did any of these things happen to you?
Month/Year

a.	Birth of a first child	1	9
b.	Became pregnant	1	9
c.	Birth of a second child	1	9
d.	Abortion	1	9

e.	Miscarriage or stillbirth	1	9
f.	Found out that cannot have children	1	9
g.	Child died	1	9

Here are some events related to *family matters*.

5. Since _____ did any of these things happen to you?
   Month/Year

a.	New person moved into household	1	9
b.	Person moved out of household	1	9
c.	Family member other than spouse or child died	1	9

Here are some events related to *where you live*.

6. Since _____ did any of these things happen to you?
   Month/Year

a.	Moved to a better residence or neighborhood	1	9
b.	Moved to a worse residence or neighborhood	1	9
c.	Built a home or had a home built	1	9
d.	Lost a home through fire, flood, or other disaster	1	9

Here are some events related to *crime and legal matters*.

7. Since _____ did any of these things happen to you, to a member of your
   Month/Year
   family, or to another person who is important to you?

		Yes		
		Yes	Important	No
		R	others	
a.	Physically assaulted or attacked	1	2	9
b.	Involved in a lawsuit	1	2	9
c.	Accused of something for which a person could be sent to jail	1	2	9
d.	Arrested	1	2	9
e.	Went to jail	1	2	9

f.	Got involved in a court case	1	2	9
g.	Convicted or found guilty of a crime	1	2	9
h.	Acquitted or found innocent of a crime	1	2	9
i.	Released from jail	1	2	9
j.	Didn't get out of jail when expected to	1	2	9

Here are some events related to *money and financial matters*.

8. Since _____ did any of these things happen to you?
   Month/Year

		Yes R	No
a.	Took out a mortgage	1	9
b.	Started buying a car, furniture, or other large purchase on the installment plan	1	9
c.	Repossession of a car, furniture, or other items bought on installment plan	1	9
d.	Took a cut in wage or salary without a demotion	1	9
e.	Suffered a financial or property loss not related to work	1	9
f.	Went on welfare	1	9
g.	Went off welfare	1	9
h.	Got a substantial increase in wage or salary without a promotion	1	9
i.	Did not get an *expected* wage or salary increase	1	9
j.	Had financial improvement not related to work	1	9

Here are some events related to *social life and recreation*.

9. Since _____ did any of these things happen to you?
   Month/Year

a.	Broke up with a friend	1	9
b.	Close friend died	1	9

Now some miscellaneous questions.

10. Since _____ did any of these things happen to you, to a member of your
       Month/Year
    family, or to another person who is important to you?

	Yes R	Yes Important others	No
a. Entered the armed services	1	2	9
b. Left the armed services	1	2	9
c. Took a trip other than a vacation trip	1	2	9

Lastly, here are some questions about *health*.

11. Since _____ did any of these things happen to you, to a member of your
       Month/Year
    family, or to another person who is important to you?

	Yes R	Yes Important others	No
a. Physical health improved	1	2	9
b. Serious physical illness started or got worse	1	2	9
c. Serious injury occurred or got worse	1	2	9

12. Did anything else important happen since _____ that I haven't
                                              Month/Year
    asked you about?

Yes	1
No	0

(If yes, ask a:)
a. What was that? (*Record verbatim and probe once for:* Did anything else important
   happen?)

Baby's Due Date _____

Baby's Birth Date _____

Goals

Your plans for when you leave here?

Stay home with baby	1
Continue with high school	2
Attend vocational/trade school	3
Attend college	4
Graduate/professional school	5
Pursue a career (obtain a job)	6

Your career goal?

Professional/technical worker	1
Manager, administrator, clerical, sales	2
Craftsman, foreman	3
Service, housekeeper, farmer, farm manager	4
Unskilled laborer	5
Not in work force	6

What steps will you take to obtain your career?

Complete high school	1
Obtain a job	2
Attend college	3
Graduate from college	4
Get a house and marry	5
Pursue a career	6

Suggestions to Others

What would you say to a girl younger than you about have a baby and the responsibility involved?

Have a baby	1
Do not have a baby	2
Do not have a baby and stay in school	3
If you have a baby, stay in school	4
Talk to others about responsibility of having a baby	5

Would you suggest she use birth control if she has a sexual relationship?

Yes	1
No	2
Say *no* to boys	3

INTERVIEWER OBSERVATIONS—TO BE COMPLETED AFTER LEAVING INTERVIEW SITE

1. *Did the respondent*

		Always	Sometimes	Never
a.	Lack interest in interview?	1	2	3
b.	Act hostile toward interviewer?	1	2	3
c.	Give answers that had little or nothing to do with questions?	1	2	3
d.	Act inappropriately cheerful?	1	2	3
e.	Cry or become tearful?	1	2	3
f.	Appear frightened or apprehensive?	1	2	3
g.	Openly lie?	1	2	3
h.	Distort facts?	1	2	3
i.	Seem uncertain?	1	2	3
j.	Answer truthfully?	1	2	3

2. *Alcohol and Drugs*

		Yes	No
a.	R drank or took drugs during interview	1	2
b.	R offered drink/drug to interviewer	1	2
c.	R's speech or manner suggested prior drinking	1	2

	Yes	No
3. Did a break-off of more than 10 minutes occur?	1	2

4. *R's grooming, personal upkeep*

Untidy, not clean	1
Average	2
Unusually clean, well groomed	3

5. Interview began _____ a.m.
p.m.

6. Interview ended _____ a.m.
p.m.

7. Location of interview _____

_____   _____
Interviewer's Signature   Date Completed

_____   _____
Supervisor's Signature   Date Reviewed

Index